ULTIMATE
BOOTY
WORKOUTS

ULTIMATE BOOTY WORKOUTS

Exercises to Build, Lift and Sculpt an Amazing Butt

Tamara Grand

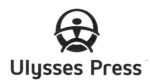

Ulysses Press

Published in the United States by
Ulysses Press
P.O. Box 3440
Berkeley, CA 94703
www.ulyssespress.com

ISBN: 978-1-61243-278-6
Library of Congress Control Number 2013947593

Printed in the United States by Bang Printing

10 9 8 7 6 5 4 3 2 1

Acquisitions: Kelly Reed
Managing editor: Claire Chun
Editors: Lauren Harrison, Lily Chou
Proofreader: Elyce Berrigan-Dunlop
Indexer: Sayre Van Young
Front cover design: what!design @ whatweb.com
Front cover images: wave graphic © Dietmar Hoepfl/shutterstock.com; woman
    © Syda Productions/shutterstock.com
Interior photographs: © Rapt Productions except page 7 women doing squats
    © Alexander Tihonov/shutterstock.com; page 14 muscle anatomy © Digital Storm/
    shutterstock.com; page 25 goblet squat © Warren Goldswain/shutterstock.com;
    page 82 hip extension © Dima Fadeev/shutterstock.com
Models: Nadia Brunner-Velasquez, Tamara Grand

Distributed by Publishers Group West

Please Note
This book has been written and published strictly for informational purposes, and in no
way should be used as a substitute for actual instruction with qualified professionals.
The author and publisher are providing you with information in this work so that you
can have the knowledge and can choose, at your own risk, to act on that knowledge.
The author and publisher also urge all readers to be aware of their health status and to
consult health care professionals before beginning any health program.

Contents

PART 1
OVERVIEW

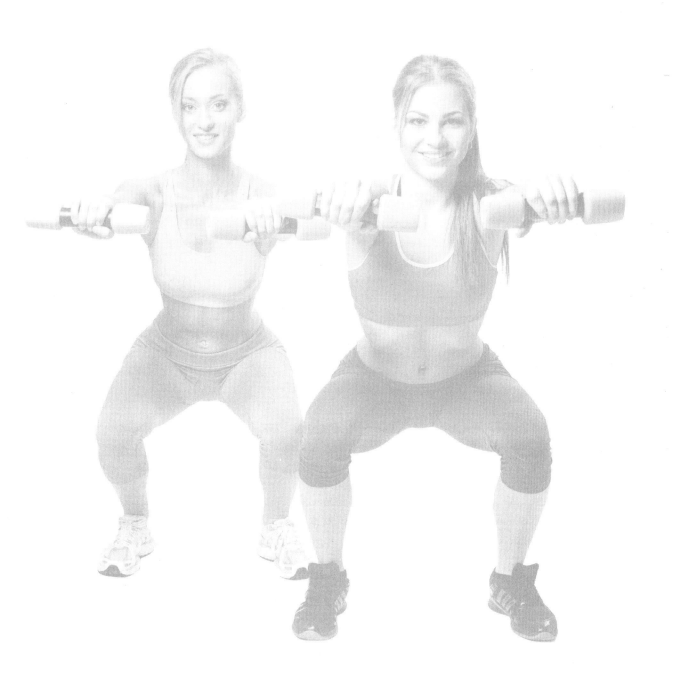

Introduction

Next to abs, butts are women's favorite thing to complain about. Too big, too flabby, too flat, too little definition, too dimpled, not enough lift. Everybody wants Beyoncé's booty, but few know what to do to get it.

The good news? Glute training is not rocket science. Combine targeted strength-training exercises with fat-melting cardio techniques and proper nutrition and you'll be on your way to the booty of your dreams in a mere 10 to 12 weeks.

A well-trained rear end isn't just nice to look at. Strong glutes and hamstrings can help improve your posture, reduce lower back, hip, and knee pain, and even reduce that stubborn abdominal "pooch." What's more, because muscle burns more calories at rest than fat does, increasing lean muscle mass via strength training can accelerate fat loss and help keep it off.

Ultimate Booty Workouts features an easy-to-follow, 12-week progressive resistance-training program designed to build and sculpt a firmer, rounder, and more muscular butt in only 30 to 40 minutes a day, 2 to 3 days a week. The workouts in this book can be done at home or at the gym with as little equipment as a few pairs of dumbbells and a stability ball. Alternative exercise options are provided for those with access to barbells, a squat rack, a cable and pulley machine, or a TRX suspension trainer.

How Glutes Training Eliminated My Lower Back Pain

In my job as a personal trainer and group fitness instructor, I spend much of my day engaged in activities that emphasize the muscles on the front of my body. After years of non-incline walking and running and teaching step aerobics and indoor cycling, I'd become "quad dominant"; the muscles on the back side of my legs were noticeably weaker than those on the front.

One day, I was teaching a small group training class how to squat on the BOSU Balance Trainer. We were using body weight only and limiting the depth to which we were squatting, an easy and familiar move for me. After completing a dozen or so repetitions, I attempted to return to standing and experienced an excruciating pain in my lower back. I couldn't straighten my upper body and carefully stepped off the BOSU. I managed to teach the remainder of the class (using verbal cues only!), but I couldn't bend over to pick weights up off the floor and had to call my husband to come and drive me home.

A trip to the physiotherapist revealed that what I'd experienced was a severe muscle spasm most likely caused by the weakness of my glutes and hamstrings as compared to my quads. A front-back muscular imbalance was causing undue strain on the muscles of my lower back, and I was given a series of glute and hamstring–strengthening exercises to perform.

Within 6 weeks of starting my "rehab" program I was not only pain-free, I was in need of a new pair of jeans. The unexpected benefit of my physiotherapist's glute-training program was a larger, higher, and firmer butt.

Today, I regularly incorporate glutes and hamstring training in my own workouts, as well as those of my group fitness classes and personal training clients. My favorite client complaint? "My butt was sore for 2 days after our last session."

About the Book

Ultimate Booty Workouts is a 12-week, progressive resistance-training program that targets the muscles of the legs, butt, and lower back. It can be used as a stand-alone program or in conjunction with your current upper-body and core-strengthening routines, depending on your fitness goals and the amount of time you have available for exercise.

The program can be completed by beginners and seasoned weight lifters alike; both basic exercises and more advanced modifications are provided for each of the three phases of the program.

The book is divided into five major sections.

PART 1 discusses the benefits of glutes training, shares tips for starting and sticking with a new exercise program, and describes the movements you'll be performing during the 12-week training program as well as the muscles behind those movements. It also provides answers to many common questions women have about strength training and offers nutritional suggestions to complement the hard work you'll be doing in the gym.

PART 2 details the 12-week program and outlines its three 4-week phases: Setting the Foundation, Building Muscle, and Leaning and Cutting. Newcomers to strength training will find definitions of common weight lifting terminology here, as well as a discussion of delayed onset muscle soreness (DOMS) and tips for measuring progress on and off the scales. Suggestions for combining this program with your existing exercise schedule are given here.

PART 3 describes and illustrates the exercises in detail. Advanced alternatives and suggestions for incorporating additional fitness tools into the workouts are also provided.

Warming up and stretching are integral parts of a successful strength training program. In **PART 4**, I discuss the elements of a good warm-up, suggest movements to warm up the muscles of the butt and legs, and provide examples of effective lower body stretches to be performed at the end of each workout. An introduction to foam rolling is also provided.

Workout templates for each of the three phases of the program can be found in the **APPENDIX**. I encourage you to make photocopies of these pages and annotate them with the details of your workouts.

Getting Ready to Move

Making the decision to start a new exercise program is easy. It's the day-to-day follow through that many people struggle with. In order to reap the benefits of *Ultimate Booty Workouts* you need to do the workout consistently, progressively, and with as much intensity as you can manage. Creating any new habit takes time and determination. Here are six tips for starting and sticking with an exercise program.

1) Create a workout schedule. Grab a calendar and plan your workouts for the next 12 weeks. You'll need to allocate 30 to 40 minutes a day, 2 to 3 days a week for the first 4 weeks, then twice per week for the remainder of the program. Always schedule at least one day off between Phase 1 and 2 workouts; 2 to 3 days of rest are recommended between the workouts in Phase 3. A Monday/Wednesday/Friday schedule works well for many people, as it leaves weekends free for other activities (or a "catch up" workout if you happen to miss one of your planned workouts for the week). Plan your workouts for times during the day when your energy is highest and you're least likely to find something "better" to do. Many people are most successful at adhering to a program when they work out first thing in the morning.

2) Announce your intentions. There's nothing like sharing your workout plan with family and friends to ensure that you get it done. Just knowing that others know you're planning on heading to the gym is a great way to stay motivated and accountable. For many, having a workout partner improves exercise adherence; it can also make exercising more fun!

3) Create a vision board. Pictures and words are powerful motivators for many. Combine photographs of fitness models whose physiques you admire with phrases that inspire and offer encouragement on a piece of poster board. Place your vision board someplace where you'll see it several times each day. If you spend a lot of time on the computer, consider scanning your vision board and using it as your computer's desktop wallpaper or screen saver.

4) Organize your gear. Whether you exercise at home or prefer to do your workouts at the gym, having your gear organized and ready to go is key to staying on track. Make sure your gym bag is always packed with clean workout clothes, running shoes, a water bottle, weight training gloves, music, a towel, your fitness journal, and a post-workout snack. Work out at home? Create a designated exercise space, a place where your equipment is always kept and with sufficient space to move about safely. Don't let lack of preparation be your excuse for missing a workout.

5) Keep track of your progress. Use a fitness journal (or photocopies of the program templates provided at the back of this book) to document your progress. Write down how many repetitions of each exercise you performed and how much weight you lifted each and every time you work out. Not only will it serve to keep track of your workout variables, thereby allowing for easier progression, a fitness journal is a great reminder of where you started and how far you've come, particularly when you're not seeing any change on the scale.

6) Celebrate "small" victories. Completed Phase 1 of the program? Increased the weight on your Squat? Mastered the Single-Leg Dead Lift? Make sure you stop and celebrate these victories. Many of my clients find that rewarding themselves for achieving small or short-term goals helps them stay motivated and focused on their programs. Think non-food rewards like pedicures, a night at the movies, or a cute new workout top, so as not to hinder your progress in the gym.

Three Moves to a Better Butt

"Train movements, not muscles." — *Vern Gambetta*

Training your glutes requires mastery of only three basic movements: hip extension, hip abduction (with and without external rotation), and knee flexion (with hips extended). Several versions of each movement are included in these workouts.

Including multiple exercises for each basic movement not only increases the number of muscle fibers stimulated during a workout (more muscle fibers means more growth), it also increases the likelihood that you're working the muscles almost to the point of fatigue or "failure," the point at which you can no longer complete another good-form repetition of the movement. In strength training, failure is success!

Below, you'll find descriptions of these three basic movements and examples of exercises used to train them.

Hip extension. Exercise physiologists define extension as any front-to-back (or "sagittal plane") movement of the body that results in the angle at a joint increasing. Hence, hips are extended when rising to standing from sitting and when reaching backward with the leg prior to kicking. We practice hip exten-sion every time we squat, lunge, perform a dead lift, and move our hips forward against gravity or external resistance. Hyperex-tension (extension beyond the normal range of motion) of the hip is also used to strengthen the lower back and upper glutes, for example during hip swings, hip thrusts, and hip extensions.

Hip abduction. Abduction is defined with respect to the midline of the body. When an arm or leg is moved away from the midline, abduction occurs. Examples of exercises involving hip abduction include Lying Leg Raises and Cable-and-Pulley Lateral Leg Raises with toes pointing forward (neutral), toward the body (internal rotation of the hip), or away from the body (external rotation of the hip).

Knee flexion. Flexion occurs in the same plane of motion

A Note about Lifting to "Failure"

In weight lifting, "failure" is defined as the point at which your muscles are physically incapable of performing another repetition of a particular exercise. Although long touted as the best way to improve strength and increase muscle mass, it's now recognized that lifting to complete muscular failure increases the potential for overtraining and psychological burnout.

Why? Routinely lifting to failure is taxing on the central nervous system and often results in sloppy, poor-form final repetitions.

Rather than push each and every set to complete muscular failure, I encourage my clients to finish their sets while they're still able to push out 1 or 2 additional good-form reps. Lifting to failure is only recommended for experienced lifters and then only during the final set of each exercise.

as extension and describes a decrease in the angle at the joint. You flex your knee by bending it. Knee flexion is controlled by muscles both above and below the knee; only those above the knee contribute directly to gluteal development. Examples of knee flexion exercises included in *Ultimate Booty Workouts* include Hamstring Curls on the Ball, Bent-Knee Dead Lifts, squats, and lunges.

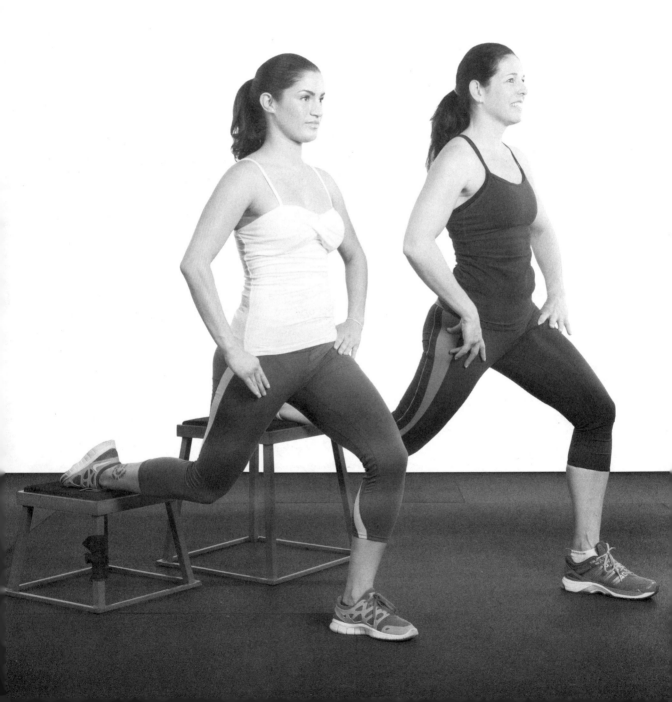

The Muscles Behind the Movement

By far the largest and potentially most powerful group of muscles in the body, the gluteals (gluteus maximus, gluteus medius, gluteus minimus) and the hamstrings (biceps femoris, semitendinosus, semimembranosus) are the primary muscles involved in the movements described above.

However, many of the exercises used in glute and hamstring training are compound in nature, meaning that they use additional muscles to assist and stabilize. In addition to building a better butt, the workouts in this book will also strengthen and help to define your thighs, calves, and core.

Gluteus maximus. The largest of the three gluteal muscles, the gluteus maximus creates the general shape of your rear end. Flat and droopy? Round and lifted? It all depends on how well developed your gluteus maximus is.

The gluteus maximus attaches to the pelvic rim at one end and broadly along the iliotibial tract at the other. Its primary function is to extend or straighten the hips, for example when returning to standing from a sitting or squatting position. It also works to externally rotate the hips and assists the glute medius and minimus in hip abduction (see page 83).

The gluteus maximus works hardest during incline walking, stair climbing, jumping, squatting, lunging, and when hyperextending the hip against resistance while standing, for example during a cable kickback.

Gluteus medius and minimus. The gluteus medius and minimus are smaller than the gluteus maximus (hence their names) and are located posteriorly, attaching the top of the hip to the femur (thigh bone). The gluteus medius sits over top of the smaller gluteus minimus.

Together, they function primarily to stabilize the hip and pelvis, in particular during walking, running, and climbing. They also work with the gluteus maximus during hip abduction, external rotation (when the leg is straight), and internal rotation (when the hip is bent).

Training the gluteus medius and minimus firms the upper part of the hips and helps to shape the thighs. Note that you can't spot-reduce fat from this area simply by performing the exercises described in this book; fat loss via cardio and clean eating are also required!

Hamstrings. The three muscles that comprise the hamstring complex are located on the back of the upper leg. They cross both the hip and the knee and as such function as both hip extensors and knee flexors.

They also control hip flexion by contracting eccentrically during the downward phase of a squat or lunge. In weight-bearing exercises, they work with the quadriceps (the large muscles of your thighs) to move the torso up and down.

Developing the hamstrings, specifically the area where they meet the gluteals, is an important part of building a better butt. The more defined the separation

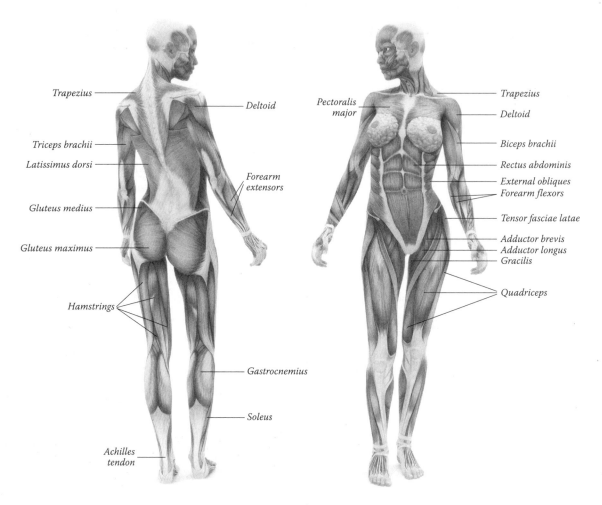

Trapezius

Deltoid

Triceps brachii

Latissimus dorsi

Forearm
extensors

Gluteus medius

Gluteus maximus

Hamstrings

Gastrocnemius

Soleus

Achilles
tendon

Pectoralis
major

Trapezius

Deltoid

Biceps brachii

Rectus abdominis

External obliques
Forearm flexors

Tensor fasciae latae

Adductor brevis
Adductor longus
Gracilis

Quadriceps

Major Muscles

between the two muscle groups, the more appealing the rear view.

As a by-product of targeted glute and hamstring training, you can also expect to see improved strength and definition in the following muscle groups:

Quadriceps. The four large muscles on the front of your thigh (rectus femoris, vastus medialis, vastus intermedius, and vastus lateralis) are collectively referred to as the quadriceps or "quads." They're responsible for knee extension and hip flexion and as such oppose the efforts of the glutes and hamstrings. When we squat or lunge, the quadriceps work on the way down (the "eccentric" phase of the exercise) and the hamstrings and glutes on the way up (the "concentric" phase of the exercise).

Calves. Two muscles on the back of the lower leg, the gastrocnemius and the soleus, assist the hamstrings in knee flexion, in particular while performing hamstring curls, but also during squats, lunges, and traditional dead lifts.

Core. When performing squats, lunges, and dead lifts with heavy weights, the deep muscles of the core assist by contracting and stabilizing the spine and torso. Posterior core muscles (erector spinae and quadratus lumborum) assist with trunk extension (for example, returning to standing at the end of a squat or dead lift), while the transverse abdominis, sitting low and deep on the front of the pelvis, compresses the abdomen during heavy exertion. While not the primary movers during glute and hamstring training, your rectus abdominis (the "six-pack" muscle) and obliques do assist in protecting the abdomen and with spinal and hip stabilization while straining and lifting.

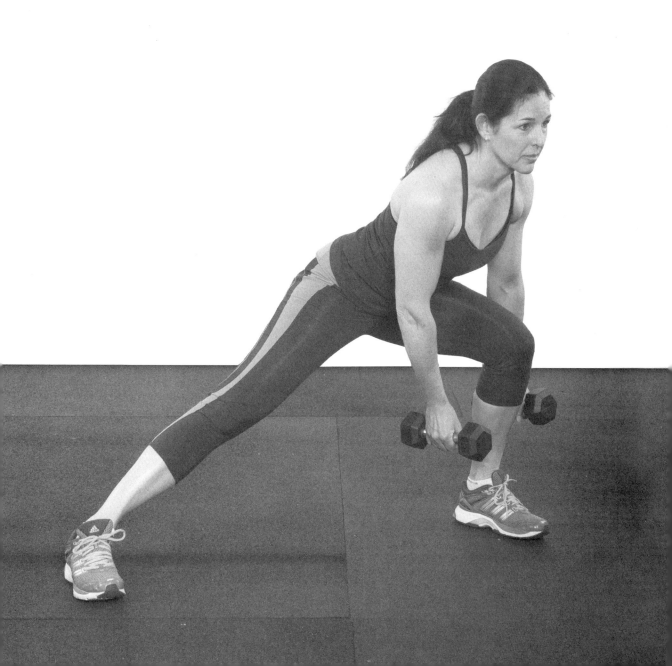

Women and Weight Lifting

Despite the wealth of information on the benefits to be gained from strength training, many women still avoid the free weights section of the gym, preferring to spend their workout time doing cardio and abdominal exercises.

While cardiovascular training is an important component of a well-balanced fitness program (and specific forms of cardio will help you shed the layer of subcutaneous fat covering the muscles beneath; see Part 2), developing and defining your glutes requires that you get comfortable lifting weights. Heavy weights.

Take a minute and think about the "weights" you lift in your everyday life: purses, laptop bags, groceries, and small (or not-so-small) children. All weigh considerably more than the "pink" dumbbells in the women's-only sections of many gyms. In order to build muscle and improve your physique, you must subject your body to heavier loads than it's already conditioned to lift.

Will you get "bulky"? Not at all. Women don't have the testosterone required to build big, bulky muscles. Lifting heavy weights will not make you look "mannish" or undermine your femininity. Think of your favorite fitness model, the one whose figure you admire and would love to have. I guarantee that she lifts heavy and often.

Women who lift weights regularly not only build shapely muscle, they also enjoy a number of health benefits, including:

Elevated rate of fat loss. Fat loss requires a daily caloric deficit. Burn more calories than you consume and you'll lose fat (and perhaps weight too; we'll talk about the difference a bit later). Unlike fat, muscle is metabolically active, meaning than even when you're not exercising, your muscles will burn calories from stored fat.

Given that the glutes and hamstrings are two of the largest muscle groups in yowur body, their potential to contribute to fat loss is not to be underestimated. Build a bigger butt and stronger legs and you're likely to drop a jeans size or two (although you may have to change your preferred cut; see page 30).

In addition, certain types of strength workouts can generate an "afterburn" effect. Technically referred to as EPOC (Excess Post-exercise Oxygen Consumption), the afterburn effect results in your body burning calories at an accelerated rate for 24 to 48 hours post-exercise. To generate an afterburn effect, your workout must be sufficiently intense so as to generate an oxygen debt. Phases 2 and 3 of the *Ultimate Booty Workouts* are designed to capitalize on the afterburn effect.

Increased bone density. Bone density peaks somewhere between 5 and 10 years after we reach skeletal maturity. From that point on, the rate at which old and damaged bone is absorbed typically exceeds the rate of new bone formation. Hence, bone density tends to decline with age and does so in three distinct phases.

The first phase starts at approximately age 30 and proceeds at a rate of 1 percent per year until menopause (complete cessation of menstruation) is reached. For about the next 5 years, the annual rate of bone density loss increases to between 2 and 3 percent. During the third phase, bone density loss slows back down to premenopausal rates. For the average woman, this translates into a loss of about 53 percent of their peak bone density by the time they reach their 80th birthday!

Reduced bone density can lead to osteoporosis, a disease that causes severe disfigurement and increased susceptibility to bone fractures.

The good news is exercises that place mechanical stress on the bones can postpone and even reverse the effects of aging on bone-density loss. Strength training, "plyometric" or jump training, and even some forms of yoga can stimulate bone growth. And the earlier you start incorporating them in your training, the greater the benefit.

Better posture. As a consequence of our modern sedentary lifestyle, many of us suffer from poor posture. Prolonged periods of sitting, either on the couch, in the car, or while working at the computer can lead to tight, shortened hip flexors and weak, over-stretched hip extensors (not to mention rounded shoulders, hunched backs, and protruding bellies). Over time, these deviations from ideal posture can become irreversible, resulting in joint pain and reduced range of motion.

Two of the most common postural deviations are swayback (characterized by an exaggerated inward curve between the pelvis and ribs) and kyphosis-lordosis (characterized by both an exaggerated curve in the lower spine and rounded, forward-sloping shoulders), can be corrected by strengthening the glutes and obliques and stretching out the opposing hip flexors.

Improving your posture via glute and hamstring training might just be the quickest way to look 5 pounds lighter and 5 years younger!

Decreased risk of injury. Strengthening muscles, bones, joints, and ligaments decreases your risk of injury both while participating in your favorite sport and during the physical activities of day-to-day life.

Many of the exercises included in the *Ultimate Booty Workouts* are functional in nature, meaning they mimic the movements that your body needs to be able to execute daily. Studies have shown that functional training not only reduces your risk of injury, it also increases joint range of motion and decreases joint pain. Squatting and lunging? Pushing and pulling? All are functional, fat-burning, booty-building movements.

Nutrition for Strength Training

Alas, no matter how hard we work to build muscles and increase strength, revealing those hard-earned muscles requires attention to diet and nutrition. Exercise is not a license to eat whatever you want—especially if great glutes are your goal.

Nutrients are the life-sustaining substances found in food. There are six major classes of nutrients (carbohydrates, protein, fat, water, vitamins, and minerals) that work together to supply your body with energy and the structural materials required to regulate growth, maintenance, and repair of the body's tissues. Because carbohydrates, protein, and fat are the most relevant nutrients to muscle building and fat loss, I discuss each in more detail below.

Carbohydrates ("carbs") are the most important nutrient for exercising muscles. Stored carbohydrates, in the form of glycogen, are the primary fuel for exercise. They are essential not only for muscular performance, but also for proper brain and central nervous system function. They help to regulate digestion by adding fiber to your diet. Contrary to popular belief, carbohydrates are not just found in breads, cereals, and pasta. Fruits, vegetables, and even dairy contribute to your daily carbohydrate intake.

Note that not all carbs are created equal. Simple carbohydrates such as baked goods, crackers, white bread, and pasta are metabolized rapidly by the body, resulting in elevated blood sugars, overproduction of insulin, and fat storage. Complex carbohydrates such as fruits, vegetables, and whole-grain breads, cereals, and pastas are always a healthier choice. Not only do they trigger less of an "insulin response," complex carbs also contain moderate amounts of several important vitamins and minerals and provide your body with the fiber it needs for proper elimination.

Protein is required to build and repair body tissue. When we fatigue our muscles by lifting heavy weights, the amino acids found in dietary protein are utilized to repair and rebuild the muscle fibers. Protein is also a major component of hormones and antibodies and hence is important for immune function and overall energy levels.

Proteins are structural molecules made up of specific combinations of 20 different amino acids, 8 of which cannot be synthesized by the body and therefore must be supplied by the diet. Animal proteins tend to be "complete" in that they provide all 20 of the required amino acids. Plant-based proteins are almost always incomplete, meaning that vegetarian and vegan athletes must include a variety of plant proteins in their diets to ensure that they're not lacking in any particular amino acid.

Fat is the chief storage form of energy in the body. Along with carbohydrates, fats are metabolized to provide your body with energy throughout the day, as well as during exercise. Dietary fats are required for the uptake

Recommended Carbohydrate Sources

Starchy complex carbohydrates will both fuel your workouts and help to replenish muscle glycogen afterward. Limit servings to ½ cup (cooked where appropriate), two to three times daily:

- Bananas
- Beans and legumes
- Brown rice
- Oats (whole or steel-cut, not instant)
- Sweet potatoes
- Whole grains (including barley, teff, and couscous)

The remainder of your daily carbohydrate intake should consist of an assortment of vegetables and fruits.

Recommended Protein Sources

Protein is the ultimate lean bodybuilding food. Aim for one 3- to 4-ounce serving at each and every meal. Note that due to their high-calorie density, the recommended serving size for all nuts and seeds is 1 ounce.

Animal protein sources:

- Bison and other game meats
- Eggs and egg whites
- Fish, shrimp, and shellfish
- Pork (leaner cuts)
- Poultry such as turkey and chicken

Plant-based alternatives:

- Beans and legumes
- Nuts and seeds (which are also healthy fats)
- Quinoa
- Tofu, tempeh, and other soy products

Recommended Fat Sources

Although our bodies need fat to perform properly, due to fat's high calorie density, limit your serving size to 1 to 2 tablespoons of oils and 1 ounce of nuts and seeds per meal. Healthy fat suggestions include:

- Avocado
- Extra-virgin olive and coconut oils
- Flax and chia seeds
- Nuts such as almonds and walnuts
- Nut butters (sugar- and salt-free, please) such as almond butter
- Pumpkin and sunflower seeds

of certain fat-soluble vitamins (vitamins A, D, E, and K) and for the proper functioning of cell membranes, skin, and hormones.

Fat is the most concentrated source of food energy, supplying more than twice as many calories by weight (9 calories per gram) as protein or carbohydrates (4 calories per gram each). Although it is calorie dense, adopting a low-fat diet in an attempt to reduce daily caloric intake often backfires. Fat makes food taste good and contributes to feelings of satiety. Often, low-fat versions of our favorite foods replace fat with sugar and sugar substitutes to make them palatable. Give me healthy fat over sucralose, aspartame, and agave nectar any day!

Ultimate Booty Workouts is an exercise program, not a menu plan. I am a personal trainer, not a dietician. Diet is a very personal thing. What works for one person doesn't always work for another. I've had clients who've lost pounds and inches by drastically reducing their carbohydrate intake. For others, that approach has led to intense cravings, sugar binges, and ultimately weight gain.

We all need to find ways to fuel our bodies that are healthy and sustainable. For some, that means eating five to six meals a day. For others, it means eliminating wheat, grains, or dairy. I encourage you to think of food as fuel and to find an approach to eating that works for YOUR body. Keeping a journal is a great tool for exploring the connection between food, performance, and physique. Try jotting down what you eat, how you feel afterward, and your energy levels before, during, and post-workout. Use this information to tweak your menu plan until you find the best dietary solution for reaching YOUR health and fitness goals.

Still stuck? Seek out the services of a registered dietician or nutritionist who specializes in sports nutrition. Have them study your food journal and create a menu plan specifically for YOUR dietary needs.

That being said, when eating for fat loss and muscle gain, the following general recommenda-tions provide a great starting point:

Eliminate processed food from your diet. If it comes in a box and has many unpronounce-able ingredients, chances are it's high in sugar, salt, and saturated fat. Real food doesn't require a nutrition label. Stick to the periphery of the grocery store; that's where you'll find the freshest and healthiest options.

Choose complex over simple carbohydrates. Whole grains, brown rice, and quinoa won't generate the same insulin response as their "white" coun-terparts. Avoid the temptation to eliminate carbohydrates entirely; they're required for the produc-tion of glycogen, which you need to help build muscle.

Eat more vegetables and fruits. Fruits and veggies are full of vitamins, nutrients, and fiber. They fill you up and are naturally low in calories. If you're concerned about fat loss, reduce your intake of starchy vegetables (potatoes, yams, and squash) and sugary fruits (watermelon, grapes, and bananas). Eat a rain-bow and experiment with differ-ent ways of cooking vegetables to keep them interesting.

Choose leaner protein sources. Fish, poultry, and eggs typically have less fat than beef or pork. Whey or vegan protein powders are a great way to fit in an extra serving of protein mid-day; use them in shakes, smooth-ies, and "cleaner" versions of your favorite pancakes and waffles. Make sure to always check the label for additives, preservatives, and artificial sweeteners; many people consider protein powder a processed food. Vegetarians can find protein in soy, beans, legumes, seeds, and nuts.

Don't skip breakfast. When it comes to changing your phy-sique, breakfast may be the most important meal of the day. Stud-ies have shown that people who eat a healthy, balanced breakfast are more successful at losing weight (and fat), than those who remain in the fasted state until mid-morning or later. Eating breakfast helps to kick-start your metabolic engine and may keep you from reaching for salty and sugary snacks later in the day.

Eat at regular intervals. Don't wait until you're starving to eat. Consuming smaller meals at regular intervals helps to stabilize blood sugars and reduce cravings for simple sugars. Experiment with the timing of your meals to see what works best for you. Many women who lift weights fol-low a three-meal and two-snack a day plan; never going more than 3 or 4 hours without food.

Combine complex carbs and protein at each and every meal. Protein takes longer to digest

Do commercially produced protein bars make a good post-workout snack?

Despite what the companies who make them would have you think, most commercially produced protein bars qualify as processed food. While a convenient and portable source of protein, many also contain added sugars (natural and artificial), preservatives, and artificial flavors, ingredients we're trying to reduce and eliminate from our *Ultimate Booty Workouts* meal plan.

Why not make your own instead? Here are two protein bar recipes that I've created to act as quick, on-the-go, post-workout snacks. Experiment with the ingredients to find a taste and texture that suits you. Make in large batches, freeze single servings, and toss in your bag before you head to the gym.

CHIA, HEMP, AND BUCKWHEAT PROTEIN BARS

2 cups ground old-fashioned oatmeal (not instant)	6 egg whites
⅓ cup buckwheat	½ cup unsweetened applesauce
⅓ cup hemp hearts	2 teaspoons vanilla extract
⅓ cup chia seeds	¼ cup honey (optional; I like them without)
1 tablespoon baking powder	¾ cup nonfat milk or unsweetened almond milk
1 teaspoon baking soda	½ cup dried cranberries
2 teaspoons ground cinnamon	½ cup chopped pecans
4 scoops protein powder (about 20 g protein per scoop)	½ cup chocolate chips (optional)

1. Preheat the oven to 350°F and line a 9 x 13-inch baking pan with parchment paper.

2. Stir together the dry ingredients in a large bowl. Whisk together the egg whites, applesauce, vanilla, honey (if using), and milk in a medium bowl.

3. Pour the wet ingredients over the dry ingredients and top with the dried fruit, nuts, and chocolate chips (if using). Stir until just combined; do not overmix.

4. Scrape batter into the prepared pan. Bake for 20 minutes. Bars will look slightly underdone when you take them out.

5. Place the pan on a cooling rack. Cool for 20 minutes, then cut into 24 equal-size bars.

Nutritional info per square (approximate): Calories, 140; Total Fat, 4.6 g; Sat. Fat, 1.1 g; Carbs, 14 g; Fiber, 2.4 g; Sugar, 4.5 g; Protein, 8 g.

PUMPKIN AND OATMEAL PROTEIN BARS

3 cups old-fashioned oats (not instant)	½ cup no-sugar-added pumpkin puree
4 scoops protein powder (about 20 g protein per scoop)	½ cup no-sugar-added applesauce
1 teaspoon ground cinnamon	¼ cup honey
½ teaspoon ground nutmeg	½ cup egg whites
½ teaspoon ground ginger	½ cup sliced almonds

1. Preheat the oven to 350°F. Line an 8 x 8-inch glass pan with parchment paper.

2. In a large bowl, combine the oats, protein powder, and spices together. In a medium bowl, whisk together the pumpkin, applesauce, honey, and egg whites together until smooth. Pour over the oat mixture and mix well. Stir in the almonds.

3. Evenly press the mixture into the prepared pan. Bake for 25 to 35 minutes, or until golden brown.

4. Cool and slice into 12 squares.

Nutritional info per square (approximate): Calories, 155; Carbohydrates, 22.3 g; Dietary Fiber, 2.8 g; Sugar, 6.7 g; Total Fat, 2.2 g; Sat. Fat, 0.2 g; Protein, 12.1 g.

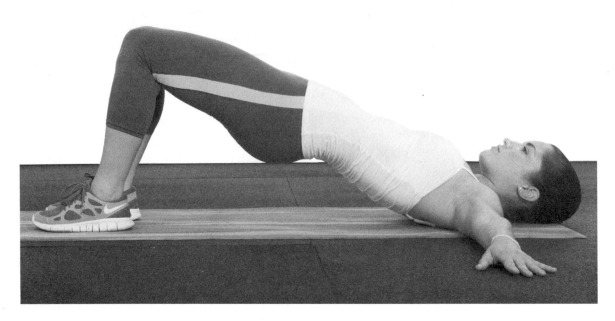

and will ameliorate the effect of carbohydrates on your blood sugars. Plus, you need the protein to support muscle growth. Many people report feeling less hungry between meals when they increase their protein intake. And swapping carbohydrates for lean protein often results in visible fat loss.

Choose healthier fats. Hydrogenated and trans fats can be avoided by simply eliminating processed foods. Choose extra-virgin olive or coconut oil over canola. Enjoy avocados, seeds, and nuts as snacks and salad toppings.

Pay attention to portion size. Even healthy foods can lead to fat storage if you eat too much of them. Aim for 3 to 4 ounces of protein and ½ to ¾ cup of complex carbohydrates at each meal.

Dietary fat is particularly calorie dense; 1 ounce of nuts or seeds is plenty. Vegetables and fruits? Consume to your heart's delight (with the emphasis on vegetables over fruits if fat loss is a goal).

Limit alcohol intake. At 7 calories per gram, alcohol is more calorie dense than carbohydrates and protein (but not fat). And frequently, having a drink or two can lower one's resolve to avoid other nutritionally bereft foods. While red wine does contain antioxidants, you can just as easily get them (and save yourself the extra calories) by eating a variety of fruits and vegetables.

Increase your intake of clear fluids. Hydration is crucial to muscle building and fat loss. Water and clear teas (both green and black) will keep you feeling full between meals and help

you maintain the energy levels required to get through your workouts. Aim for a minimum of eight to ten 8-ounce glasses daily. You can tell that you're properly hydrated if your urine is light in color and you need to urinate every hour or two. Avoid waiting until late in the day to drink your quota unless you enjoy middle-of-the-night trips to the bathroom.

Avoid severe caloric restriction. Low-calorie diets (fewer than 1200 calories per day for an average woman) don't provide your body with enough energy to conduct its daily tasks, never mind the high-intensity workouts described in this book. Building muscle requires fuel. Focus less on the caloric content of your meals and more on the types and amounts of nutrients you're consuming.

Fuel your body before you workout. Most people find that their workouts suffer if they haven't eaten first. Every time I've had a client complain of dizziness or nausea mid-session, lack of food has been the culprit. What and when to eat before a workout is a personal decision. My preference is always to have a combination of complex carbohydrates and lean protein (for example, eggs and whole grain toast or Greek yogurt and fruit) about 90 minutes before a workout. Experiment to find what works best for you.

Replenish glycogen by eating after exercise. Muscle glycogen is the preferred fuel for strength training. A moderate to intense workout will typically deplete glycogen stores. In the absence of post-workout refueling, glycogen recovery can take up to 24 hours. Studies have shown that you can speed up the rate of glycogen resynthesis by consuming carbohydrates and a small amount of protein within an hour or two of your workout. My post-workout snack of choice? Whey protein blended with berries, spinach, and unsweetened almond milk: portable, filling, and quick to drink.

A Few Words About Cellulite...

You're probably familiar with cellulite: the dimpled-looking fat stores that tend to accumulate on the legs and buttocks of most adult females. Cellulite is caused by "herniation" of the fat within the body's fibrous connective tissues. Essentially, it's fat that has escaped the tissues that normally contain it. Regardless of what causes it, most women wish it would go away.

It's partly genetic, meaning that if your mother had notice-able cellulite, chances are you will as well. But it's also affected by hormones, nutrition, and exercise. Contrary to the promises of late night television infomercials and the ads that line the margins of most fitness magazines, there is no scientifically based cure for cellulite.

One can, however, make it less noticeable by reducing overall body fat and "plumping" up the underlying muscle via strength training. Flattering clothing and a bit of a tan can help too.

While I make no promises that your cellulite will disappear after completion of the *Ultimate Booty Workouts* program, many of my female clients report visible reductions in the appearance of cellulite after following the strength training programs I design for them and dialing in their nutrition by eliminating added sugar and processed foods.

PART 2
THE PROGRAM

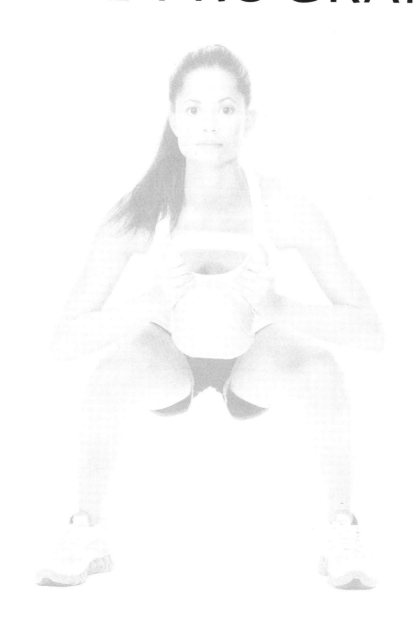

How to Use This Book

Ultimate Booty Workouts is a 12-week training program consisting of three distinct, 4-week phases: Setting the Foundation, Building Muscle, and Leaning and Cutting.

For each phase, I provide exercise options for Beginners (no experience with strength training), Intermediate (less than a year's experience with strength training but competent at squatting, lunging, and performing dead lifts), and Advanced exercisers (more than a year's experience in the gym and comfortable with using heavy loads).

Just because you start a phase with the Beginner moves doesn't mean that you won't progress to the Intermediate moves by the end of the month. As discussed below, progression is integral to getting results in the gym. Note that some movements will be easier to advance than others. For example, I tend to be able to progress my glute exercises more quickly than those targeting my hamstrings.

Veteran gym-goers may be tempted to skip Phase 1 and dive right into the Phase 2 workouts. However, even "regulars" in the weight room can benefit from analyzing their exercise form and concentrating on improving their range of motion with slower lifts and lighter loads. Skip Phase 1 at your peril!

During Phase 1 you'll be Setting the Foundation: learning to "turn on" and engage your gluteal and core muscles. Practice your squats, lunges, and dead lifts first with body weight and then with as much load as you can handle while still maintaining good form over the prescribed repetition range. Plan on two to three workouts per week, with a lower-body rest day (the importance of rest will be discussed further, later in the chapter) between workouts.

Phase 2 is all about Building Muscle (also referred to as the Hypertrophy phase). Although you'll be performing many of the same exercises as in Phase 1, you'll be using heavier weights and lowering the repetition range to keep your muscles guessing. You'll also start incorporating cardio intervals at the end of your strength session to elevate your calorie burn and help promote shedding of the layer of subcutaneous fat hiding those developing muscles. Perform the workout two times each week, with at least 48 hours rest between.

Phase 3 pairs hypertrophy training with Tabata intervals—the perfect combination for Leaning and Cutting. Again, you'll be performing fewer repetitions per set than during the previous phase, but lifting heavier and cycling between two different programs to ensure adequate rest and recovery between workouts. Plan on doing only two of these workouts per week, with at least 72 hours rest between.

Detailed descriptions of each of the three phases' workouts are described later in the chapter with suggestions for how to combine them with your regular strength and/or cardiovascular workouts.

Consistency & Progression: Two Keys to Success

"We are what we repeatedly do. Excellence, then, is not an act but a habit." —*Aristotle*

Want to see results from your efforts in the gym? Aim for consistency and progression.

This is a short-term, narrowly focused exercise program. Each phase consists of only 8 to 12 workouts. Missing just one or two workouts per phase is tantamount to missing 10 percent of the entire program. Catching up on missed workouts one week by adding extra workouts the following week will undermine your quest for a more muscular and defined derriere. It will also put you at risk of succumbing to the symptoms of overtraining: fatigue, strength plateaus, and even weight gain.

Not only will being consistent with your workouts result in a more sculpted and lifted rear end, it will also help to stabilize your blood sugars, reduce delayed onset muscle soreness (DOMS; see page 29), and make regular exercise a part of your long-term lifestyle.

Muscular fitness is developed by placing a demand, or overload, on the muscles in a manner to which they are not already accustomed. Slowly increasing the overload over time (known as "progressive resistance training") is the key to building muscles and increasing both muscular strength and endurance. Gradually increasing intensity also reduces the likelihood of injury.

General guidelines for increasing load are to not increase weight by more than 10 percent at a time. I also recommend not increasing the load (or progressing to a more advanced

---

Gym Etiquette 101

New to exercising in a gym? Follow these guidelines to ensure a safe and enjoyable workout (and to ensure the safety, enjoyment, and consideration of your fellow gym-goers).

- Wear proper gym attire, including footwear

- Avoid "sharing" your musical tastes with others; set the volume on your music player so that only you can hear it

- If you don't know how to operate equipment, ask an attendant

- Pay attention to the people around you, in particular those moving heavy loads

- Don't hog the equipment; let others "work in" if you're resting between sets

- Put dumbbells, barbells, and other tools back where they belong when you're finished with them

- Wipe down all machines and equipment after use

---

version of an exercise) on more than one or two exercises each workout.

Equipment Requirements

While the workouts in this book can be performed at home, most home gyms don't have the heavy equipment that you'll require as you progress through the program. By the eighth or tenth week, 10-, 15-, and even 20-pound dumbbells won't be heavy enough to fatigue your muscles by the end of the specified repetition range. If a long-term gym membership isn't in your budget, consider signing up for just a month or two. Many gyms will give you 30 days for next to nothing as a way to entice you to purchase another

11 months. Be warned, though—strength training is addictive, and you just may not want to give up that membership when the month ends!

If you decide to train at home, you'll need to have the following pieces of equipment at your disposal:

Three or four sets of dumbbells, in 5-pound increments. Even if you're an absolute beginner, don't start with anything lighter than 10 pounds. None of the exercises in this program require you to lift the weights above shoulder height, and if you regularly carry groceries, laundry baskets, or children, your lower body will already be adapted to lifting loads in the 10 to 40 pound range. My recommendation?

Start with 10s, 15s, and 20s, and be prepared to purchase additional pairs of dumbbells as you get stronger. Consider investing in a set of nested or interchangeable weights (well-known brands include Bowflex and Power-Block); they take up less space and are more economical than multiple pairs of dumbbells.

A step, bench, plyo box, or sturdy ottoman (12 to 18 inches in height). A flat, weight-training bench is the best, but also the priciest option. Step aerobics benches with extra risers can sometimes be purchased online or at big-box fitness stores for $30 to $40. In a pinch, a heavy ottoman (placed against a wall to reduce the likelihood of it slipping) can also be used. Check out websites like craigslist.com for affordable, preowned exercise benches and equipment.

A stability or physiotherapy ball. Stability balls come in three sizes: 55, 65, and 75 cm. The taller you are, the larger the ball you'll need. I generally recommend that women between 5'4" and 5'8" purchase a 65 cm ball. Taller than 5'8"? Purchase the largest size. Not quite 5'4"? The 55 cm ball will suit you perfectly.

A yoga or Pilates mat. These can be purchased just about anywhere, including sporting goods stores, pharmacies, book stores, and department stores.

The equipment listed below is not required, but strongly recommended. It will allow you to incorporate more variety in your workouts and can be used to build upper-body strength as well. Most can be found at commercial gyms, with the exception of the TRX (although this is changing as it increases in popularity and becomes more readily available):

Barbells, bars, and weight plates. If you have a squat rack, then you'll definitely want to invest in an Olympic bar and

Using an Olympic Bar

Using an Olympic bar requires extra precautions:

Before starting your set, place the Olympic bar supports at a height such that you have to duck slightly to set the bar across your shoulders. If the supports are placed too high, it's difficult (and dangerous) to "rack" the bar at the end of your set.

If you're new to using the O-bar, or attempting a heavy load for the first time, make sure that the horizontal safety bars are also in place. Setting them at pelvis height will allow you to "drop" the bar safely, if you've chosen too heavy a weight and can't complete the lift.

Load the bar with plates, making sure that the load is equal on both sides. Use clips to secure your plates, even if you're only using 5 or 10 pounds.

Many gyms have a padded cushion that you can place around the bar to reduce pressure on the back of your shoulders. Don't be afraid to use it; even the big guys like a little comfort in the gym.

Start each set by standing in front of the bar, with your feet hip-distance apart or slightly wider.

Step back until the bar is just touching your shoulders. Place your hands on the bar, well outside your shoulders, with palms facing forward. Pull your shoulder blades back and down, creating a ledge for the bar (and padded cushion, if you're using one) to rest upon. Bend your knees and lower your torso slightly so that you're standing directly under the bar. Extend your legs to rise to standing with the bar across your shoulders. Step back from the bar supports. Complete all reps (as described for the Barbell Back Squat).

After you've completed the exercise, step forward until the bar is resting on the bar supports; don't let go until you've visually confirmed that both sides of the bar are secure! Step out from under the bar.

At the end of your last set, return the weight plates to their proper storage place; nobody likes to have to unload the previous user's plates before they start their own workout.

weight plates. At 45 pounds "naked," it's the best tool out there for upping the weights on your squats and dead lifts. No rack? Try a shorter, EZ-curl bar with weight plates and clips. The bar itself weighs 22.5 pounds and plates can be purchased (always in pairs) in 5-pound increments.

Kettlebells. Kettlebell swings are one of the best exercises for developing strong glutes. They're also great for engaging your core and elevating your heart rate. While dumbbells and SandBells can be used in their place, most people find the kettlebell to be more ergonomic.

TRX Suspension Trainer. Suspension trainers are a wonderful, whole-body training tool that require nothing more than a secure anchor point and your body weight. I like using them for single-leg exercises, in particular when teaching clients how to perform Single-Leg Squats. They're also great for making Rear-Foot Elevated Lunges more difficult and increasing the recruitment of deep-core stabilizer muscles while training glutes and legs. Plus, the TRX packs up into a stuff-sack small enough to fit in your suitcase; no more missing workouts while on vacation!

Before You Begin

The exercises in *Ultimate Booty Workouts* have been designed to physically challenge the muscles of your lower body. While strenuous exercise can help to improve overall health, if you are pregnant or have high blood pressure, a heart condition, diabetes, or suffer from joint pain or osteoarthritis, you should seek your doctor's permission before beginning this or any other fitness program.

Always modify exercises to suit your own physical abilities and fitness level. Never, ever work through pain: physical pain is the body's way of telling you to stop before further injury occurs. Some of the most common injuries associated with strength training are strains, sprains, and dislocations (although bruised shins from heavy dead lifts may occur too).

Treat strains and sprains with rest, ice, compression, and elevation (RICE). You may find that you need a few extra days of rest before resuming your workouts. Ibuprofen can also help reduce inflammation and swelling. Dislocations are very rarely experienced with lower-body training; however, if you suspect a knee, ankle, or hip dislocation, see your doctor or physiotherapist immediately.

When lifting weights, it's important to recognize the difference between pain and discomfort. While we try our best to avoid pain, discomfort is strongly encouraged! Discomfort during the workout, for example, the burning sensation you experience near the end of a set of heavy squats, is merely an indication that your muscles are nearing fatigue and that you're challenging yourself appropriately. Get comfortable with discomfort; that's where physical change begins.

Sometimes muscles are stiff and sore a day or two after a particularly challenging workout. Mild delayed onset muscle soreness (DOMS) is nothing to be concerned about; in fact, it indicates that your muscles were taxed enough during the previous workout to induce repair and growth. You can help reduce the intensity of DOMS by performing some light cardiovascular exercise after your strength-training session and finishing up with some foam rolling and an extended stretch (see Part 4 for foam rolling tips and stretching ideas).

If, however, DOMS lasts more than 3 days or is so intense that it makes climbing stairs and getting up from the toilet difficult, you need to reduce the intensity of your workouts just a bit. While it might seem that longer-lasting discomfort is an indicator that you're "pushing it" and making progress in the gym, extended

DOMS is actually counterproductive. You're more likely to miss a workout or two while you recover, thereby undermining your longer-term strength goals. (Note that the Phase 3 shift toward focusing on the eccentric part of each contraction will tend to increase the intensity of DOMS.)

Tips for Measuring Progress

While weight loss is often the primary goal for starting an exercise program, when working to build muscle there are better tools for measuring progress than your bathroom scale.

Because muscle is denser than fat, pound for pound, it takes up less space in your body. When you simultaneously lose fat and gain muscle (as you will on this program), weight loss can be slow or even nonexistent. Rather than focusing on body weight as an indicator of progress, try one of the following:

Measure yourself. At the beginning of each of the three phases of the program, grab a measuring tape and measure your chest (nipple height), abdomen (belly button height), hips (widest part around your butt), and thighs (right and left, at the very, very top). If you're losing fat and gaining muscle, you're likely to see the first two decrease. Hips and thighs can go either way,

depending on how quickly your body is able to put on muscle. Hint, if all four measurements increase, it's more likely to be fat than muscle and you need to critically examine your diet. Go back to Part 1 and have another read through Nutrition for Strength Training (page 18).

Take a picture. Before and after shots don't lie. Because we see ourselves in the mirror many times each day, it's difficult to recognize changes in our own physiques. At the same time that you measure yourself, take three photos, one each from the front, back, and side. Wear close-fitting exercise clothes and if possible, wear the same clothes for each photo shoot.

Try on your favorite jeans. Whether they fit perfectly now or are a bit too small, these jeans will be your truest indicator of the changes that are taking place in your body. As you become leaner and more muscular, they'll fit you differently and you may just find yourself looking to replace them at the end of the 12-week program. Note, however, that many women who train their glutes regularly find that the cut of jeans they wore previously no longer flatters their higher, firmer derriere. Celebrate by experimenting with a new style or two.

Journal your workouts. Keeping a detailed workout journal is the best way to gauge your progress. Write down your reps, sets, and weights each time you work out. Not only will it make it easier to remember when it's time to progress an exercise (more on that below), it will also show you how far you've come in a relatively short period of time. Check out the Appendix for program templates that you can photocopy and take with you to the gym.

Combining the Ultimate Booty Workouts with Your Regular Exercise Program

For the next 12 weeks, your primary workout focus will be on developing the muscles of your legs and rear end.

If you're currently doing whole-body training or body-part splits, you'll need to reorganize your training schedule to accommodate the workouts described in this book. Resist the temptation to try and do it all; working glutes and hamstrings via whole-body training on your "rest" days will undermine the effects of the glute and leg-focused workouts.

With strength training, less is often more.

Similarly, performing too much cardiovascular training, in particular, long, slow distance or endurance training, can negatively impact lower-body strength gains. Not only will it fatigue the muscles you need to squat, lunge, and dead lift heavy, it may also counteract the metabolism-boosting effects of the *Ultimate Booty Workouts*. We all know women who decide to train for their first half or full marathon in an attempt to lose weight and "get fit." In most cases, despite the overwhelming volume of training they've done, their bodies look almost the same after the event as they did when they were only running a mile or two a week. Endurance cardio only makes you better at endurance cardio.

For each of the 3 phases of the program, I've included specific instructions for cardiovascular training that will enhance the effects of the leg and glutes workouts. If you just can't refrain from adding extra cardio, try limiting it to a maximum of 30 minutes, once or twice a week, and performing it either after your lower-body workout or on a day when you're not training legs and glutes.

Adding daily, low-intensity walks to your schedule is a great way to (1) aid muscular recovery, (2) reduce your body's production of stress hormones (which results in abdominal fat deposition), and (3) accumulate enough daily steps for optimal health.

On the Importance of Rest

Often when we start a new exercise program, our excitement to see results leads to doing too much, too soon. Not only does lifting too frequently increase your risk of injury, it can also undermine your strength and endurance gains.

Every time we perform an exercise to near-fatigue, we're creating micro tears in the tendons, ligaments, and muscles themselves. It's the repair and rebuilding process that makes muscles bigger and stronger, allowing us to lift heavier the next time we hit the gym.

Most fitness professionals recommend resting a muscle group for 24 to 72 hours between workouts; the more intense the workout, the longer the prescribed rest period. You'll notice that my suggested rest period between workouts increases from 48 hours in Phase 2 to 72 hours in Phase 3. That's because Phase 3 workouts are significantly more challenging than those in Phase 2.

Do you need to spend your "rest day" on the couch watching sitcom re-runs? Not at all! Train a different muscle group or enjoy a day of "active recovery"; walk, cycle, hike, sail, kayak, golf, or attend a yoga class. Use your rest day to enjoy your favorite non-gym activity.

Many of the exercises described in this book simultaneously work your glutes, legs, and core. For example, Single-Leg Dead Lifts require strong stabilization from your obliques and erector spinae. One of the benefits of glutes training is a stronger, more stable midsection. That being said, you may still wish to add an extra day (or two) of targeted core training if you're looking for six-pack abs as well as a better booty.

Below are two suggestions for combining the *Ultimate Booty Workouts* with your regular upper-body and core strength training workouts. Remember that glutes and leg training is your priority for the next 12 weeks; everything else is subject to how much time and energy you have for additional workouts.

Perform your upper-body strength workouts on your leg-and-glutes rest days. This approach works well if short, near-daily workouts fit with your schedule. In Phase 1, an alternating-day program might look something like this: Monday—legs and glutes, Tuesday—upper body, Wednesday—legs and glutes, Thursday—upper body, Friday—legs and glutes OR core (depending on whether you're following a 2-per-week or 3-per-week program), Saturday and Sunday—rest (see "On the Importance of Rest").

Perform upper- and lower-body strength workouts on the same day. Legs and glutes before arms, please, when your muscle glycogen levels are highest and you're feeling most energetic. You may find that you need to shorten your upper body workout to fit it all into a single session.

Hint: Choose compound exercises, low repetitions, and heavier weights for your upper-body work to avoid spending all day in the gym. For example push-ups, pull-ups, and bent-over rows. If you choose this option, make sure you're including an extra core workout, preferably on a non-strength-training day. In Phase 1, for example, you might train upper and lower body on Monday, Wednesday, and Friday (if you're performing 3 workouts each week) and train your core on Tuesday or Thursday.

Definitions of Key Terminology

Strength training has a language all its own. Here are some of the more common terms that you'll want to familiarize yourself with before starting the program.

Repetitions or "reps." The number of times you'll perform a specific exercise without taking a break. For the workouts described in this book, you'll be performing between 6 and 15 reps, depending on the exercise and the phase of the program you're in.

Sets. The number of times you'll perform the designated repetitions of a specific exercise. For example, "2 sets of 15 repetitions" means that you'll perform 15 repetitions of the exercise, rest for the amount of time indicated, then perform another 15 repetitions before moving on to the next exercise.

Superset. A pair of exercises that are performed alternately for the designated number of repetitions and sets. For example, "superset 10 repetitions of squats and dead lifts for 3 sets" means that you'll perform 10 squats, followed immediately by 10 dead lifts, followed immediately by 10 squats, etc., until 3 sets of each exercise have been completed.

Isolation exercise. An exercise that requires only a single joint or muscle group to execute. For example, a cable kickback requires only that the glutes extend (or slightly hyperextend) the hips. Isolation exercises are frequently used to rehab injured muscles or to target the weakest link in a muscular chain. Isolation exercises are best placed near the end of a workout.

Compound exercise. An exercise that requires multiple joints and muscle groups to execute. For example, squat-ting requires flexion of the hips, knees, and ankles, and simultaneously recruits the glutes, hamstrings, and quads. Compound exercises tend to be more metabolic than isolation exercises are, although both have their place in body-part-specific training. Begin your workout with compound exercises.

Concentric contraction. A contraction in which the muscle exerts force, shortens, and over-comes resistance. Also called the "working phase of the exercise." For example, when performing a hamstring curl, the hamstring contracts concentrically to flex the knee against resistance.

Eccentric contraction. A contraction in which the muscle exerts force, lengthens, and is overcome by resistance. Also called the "non-working" phase of an exercise. In the above described hamstring curl, the hamstring can be made to work eccentrically by slowing down the return phase of the exercise. Used sparingly, eccentric training can be a great tool for overcom-ing strength plateaus (but is also known to exacerbate delayed onset muscle soreness).

Circuit training. Circuit training is essentially a long superset. A circuit might consist of 6, 8, or even 10 exercises per-formed one after the other, with little rest in between. Circuits can be timed (you perform as many repetitions of each exercise as you can within a specified time interval) or not (you perform the number of repetitions indicated, for each exercise, regardless of how long it takes you). When you complete a circuit, take a short break and begin again until you've finished the number of sets (or rounds, as they're specifically called in this type of training) required.

High-intensity interval training (HIIT). High-intensity interval training can take many forms. At its most general, it describes a method of training where specified periods of movement (either strength or cardiovascular training) are alternated with specified periods of rest or recovery. HIIT is a great way to push yourself out of your comfort zone, increase your aerobic capacity, and elevate both your heart rate and your calorie burn during your workout. Some forms of HIIT can also generate an "afterburn" effect—the increased burning of calories for a period of 24 to 36 hours post workout. We'll be incorporating HIIT cardio intervals into our Phase 2 workouts.

Tabata training. Tabata intervals are a specific form of HIIT training. They were named after Dr. Izumi Tabata, the lead author of a study comparing the fitness benefits of a wide variety of high-intensity interval protocols. Of all the interval protocols compared, Tabata intervals resulted in the greatest improvements in aerobic conditioning, athletic performance, fat loss, and anaerobic threshold. Requiring only 4 minutes of your time, (one "Tabata" consists of 8 rounds of 20 seconds of maximal effort followed by 10 seconds of recovery), Tabata intervals are a great bang-for-your-buck addition to your regular workout. They'll make an appearance in the Phase 3 workouts.

Tips for Getting the Most Out of Your Strength Workouts

I know, you're ready to see what the workouts look like. But before we get there, I want to share with you just a few tips for getting the most out of the workouts you'll be doing for the next 12 weeks and beyond.

Tempo. When we lift weights, we subject our muscles to tension. The longer the muscles experience that tension, the greater the stimulation to grow. The more rapidly you perform an exercise, the more likely it is that you're using momentum rather than muscle. Avoid the temptation to rush through each repetition of an exercise, thinking that faster is better. Count

2 or 3 "one-thousands" for both the "working" and the "non-working" phases of the exercise. For example, take 2 to 3 seconds to lower your backside toward the floor during a squat and another 2 to 3 seconds to press back up to standing. But take care not to rest at the end of the eccentric (non-working) phase of the movement. Resting between repetitions will lead to little to no gains in strength.

Varying the tempo of a workout is also a great way to keep your muscles guessing. In Phase 3, I describe an alternate tempo that can be used by intermediate and advanced lifters to keep their muscles "guessing" and further increase their strength gains.

Range of motion (ROM). Range of motion describes the angle through which a joint allows its segments to move and varies from person to person depending on skeletal structure and flexibility. As a consequence of taking your time with each repetition, you'll be more likely to perform the movement through its entire range of motion and thereby maximize the number of muscle fibers recruited. Pay special attention to the ROM reminders given with the exercise descriptions in Part 3 of this book.

Breathing. It's not uncommon to see people holding

their breath during challenging exercises. Much of the time this is subconscious. It's important to breathe during exercise, as working muscles require oxygen to perform. Focus on breathing out (exhaling) during the working (or concentric) phase of each exercise and breathing in (inhaling) during the returning (or eccentric) phase. For example, inhale as you lower your butt toward the ground during a squat and exhale (forcefully, if you find this helps) as you push through your heels to return to standing. If you forget when you're supposed to breathe during a lift, use the phrase "whistle while you work" as a reminder.

Rating of Perceived Exertion (RPE). In the past, fitness professionals have recommended that exercisers keep their heart rate within a specified "training zone" to maximize the benefits of their workout. Rather than focus on heart rate, I prefer my clients to use the Rating of Perceived Exertion (RPE) scale. On a scale of 0 (sleeping) to 10 (impending heart attack), strength training should produce an RPE somewhere between 5 and 7. Your heart rate should be elevated above pre-workout levels, but not so high that you can't maintain a conversation (or at least a sentence or two of a conversa-

tion) while working out, and you should definitely be sweating. During HIIT and Tabata intervals, increase your RPE to 8 or 9.

Mind-to-muscle connection. Studies have shown that simply visualizing a muscle working can lead to small, but measurable increases in muscle size and strength. As you perform each exercise, concentrate on the muscles that you're working. Creating a strong mind-to-muscle connection not only improves the coordination of your lifts, it can also reduce the likelihood of injury. Save grocery list making and chatting with your workout partner for when you're stretching afterward.

Muscular fatigue or "failure." Local muscular fatigue, or failure, describes the point at which you can no longer execute another good-form repetition of a particular exercise. In progressive resistance training, "failure is success." Lifting to near-failure (as defined above) is the quickest way to see a return on your efforts in the gym. Note that adding extra, poor-form repetitions can be taxing on the central nervous system and ultimately undermine your performance and strength gains. I encourage you to always choose a weight that will almost fatigue your muscles by the end of the specified rep range. If you

can easily perform 15 repetitions of an exercise that only required 10, it's time to increase the load or choose a more challenging version of the exercise (see my earlier comments about consistency and progression, page 26).

Work your weaker side first. Most of us have noticeable left-right muscular imbalances. Our dominant side, the side we kick, throw, and write with, is almost always stronger than our non-dominant side. When performing exercises that are executed separately on each side of the body ("unilateral" exercises, like stationary lunges, for example), most of us unconsciously start with our dominant side. In doing so, we not only run the risk of being too tired to perform the last few reps on the non-dominant side (the second side is always more challenging regardless of which side we start on), we also let our stronger side dictate the weight (or exercise progression) used. Over time, this practice will exacerbate left-right weaknesses. Try starting all unilateral exercises in the *Ultimate Booty Workouts* on your non-dominant side, with the long-term goal of reducing the strength differential over time.

Phase 1: Setting the Foundation

The first 4 weeks of the program consist of a circuit-style workout.

After a short warm-up (see Part 4), perform 12 to 15 repetitions of each exercise, in the order specified, with 30 to 60 seconds rest between exercises. Once you've finished the last exercise, rest for 1 to 2 minutes before repeating the entire circuit once (Beginners) or twice more (Intermediate and Advanced exercisers). Note: If you're brand new to strength training, begin with a single cycle of the circuit. Increase to 2 cycles in the second or third week of the program.

Options for each exercise are listed in order of increasing difficulty in the chart below and described in detail in Part 3 of this book.

Do this workout one, two, or three times (maximum) per week, with at least 1 day of lower-body rest between workouts. Many of my clients see significant improvement in this phase of the program without performing any cardiovascular training at all. If you feel the need to add cardio to your routine (for many, cardiovascular training is a stress releaser), limit it to once or twice a week, for a maximum of 30 minutes.

At the end of each workout, spend 5 to 10 minutes foam rolling and stretching the muscles that you've just worked. Both are important for improving flexibility and joint ROM, as well as reducing the intensity of DOMS. See Part 4 for foam rolling tips and stretching suggestions.

When the weight (or exercise option you've chosen) is no longer heavy enough to lead to muscular near-failure by the end of the final set, either increase your load (by no more than 10%) or choose a more challenging version of the exercise. Aim to progress in one or two exercises each time you do the workout. Note that when you make an exercise more difficult, it's unlikely that you'll initially be able to perform 15 good-form repetitions. Over the next few workouts, gradually increase your reps from 12 to 15 before progressing the exercise again by moving to the next level or adding weight.

If at the end of 4 weeks, you feel that you're not quite ready to move on to Phase 2, simply extend Phase 1 for an extra week or two. We all make progress at different rates and there's no benefit to moving on to the next phase of the program before you've created a solid strength-training foundation.

Note that you don't need to have reached the most challenging version of each exercise before advancing to Phase 2.

Phase 1: Setting the Foundation

Start with a 5- to 10-minute, whole-body warm-up (page 96) and finish with foam rolling and stretching (page 104).

EXERCISE	REPS	SETS	REST
1. *Beginner:* Ball Squat p. 45 *Intermediate:* Bodyweight Squat p. 47 *Intermediate/Advanced:* Dumbbell Squat p. 47 *TRX Option:* TRX Squat p. 51	12–15	2–3	30–60 seconds
2. *Beginner/Intermediate:* Stationary Lunge p. 56 *Intermediate/Advanced:* Back Lunge p. 57	12–15 each side	2–3	30–60 seconds
3. *All levels:* Hamstring Curl on the Ball p. 63 *Intermediate/Advanced:* Bent-Leg Dumbbell Dead Lift p. 67 *TRX Option:* TRX Hamstring Curl p. 65	12–15	2–3	30–60 seconds
4. *Beginner/Intermediate:* Plié Ball Squat p. 46 *Intermediate/Advanced:* Goblet Squat p. 48	12–15	2–3	30–60 seconds
5. *Beginner:* Lateral Band Walk p. 60 *Intermediate/Advanced:* Dumbbell Lateral Lunge p. 61	12–15 each side	2–3	30–60 seconds
6. *Beginner:* Basic Glute Bridge p. 72 *Intermediate/Advanced:* Feet-Elevated Glute Bridge p. 72 *Advanced:* Weighted Glute Bridge p. 72	12–15	2–3	30–60 seconds
7. *Beginner:* Forearm Plank on Knees p. 76 *Intermediate/Advanced:* Forearm Plank on Toes p. 77	hold on as long as possible	2–3	60 seconds
Beginner: Do 2 sets in total *Intermediate/Advanced:* Do 3 sets in total			

Phase 2: Building Muscle (Hypertrophy)

In Phase 2, we'll be switching to supersets, using heavier weights and performing fewer repetitions than during Phase 1. This keeps your muscles guessing and helps to prevent strength-training plateaus.

Complete the warm-up described in Part 4, then perform 10 to 12 repetitions of each exercise, in each exercise pair. For example, the first superset in the workout is a squat/dead lift pair. Perform 10 to 12 squats, immediately followed by 10 to 12 dead lifts.

Beginners will perform two sets of each exercise pair; Intermediate and Advanced lifters will perform 3 sets. Once all sets and reps of an exercise pair are complete, move on to the next pair. Minimize rest time between exercises and exercise pairs for best results; 15 to 30 seconds should suffice.

Do this workout twice per week, attempting to progress at least one exercise each time you hit the gym. As with the workouts in Phase 1, feel free to extend Phase 2 for an additional week or more if you're not quite ready to move on to the more challenging exercises in Phase 3.

Again, it's not necessary that you've progressed to the most advanced version of every exercise before starting Phase 3, only that you've consistently increased the challenge of your workouts over the 4 weeks.

Those of you with fat-loss goals will also be adding a short High-Intensity Interval Training (HIIT) cardio workout after the weights. Note that this "finisher" is optional and can be skipped if losing fat is not a priority for you. Otherwise, continue on with your cool-down, foam rolling, and stretching, as in Phase 1.

Optional HIIT Instructions

HIIT can be performed on your favorite cardio machine, the local track, or even a long set of stairs (the best booty building cardio there is!). If you're competent with a jump rope, skipping makes for a great HIIT workout.

Beginners will alternate 30 seconds of high-intensity movement with 90 seconds of low-intensity, or recovery movement, for a total of 10 minutes (or 5 cycles). Note that high intensity implies that you're pulling out all the stops (RPE equal to 8 or 9). Depending on your fitness level, high intensity on the treadmill might vary from a 4 mph jog to a 10 mph sprint. If you can maintain your speed and intensity for longer than 30 seconds, you're not working hard enough.

Intermediate and Advanced exercisers may shorten the recovery period to 60 seconds or even 30 seconds, thereby increasing the number of cycles performed during the final 10 minutes of the workout.

Every second workout, all levels of exercisers will add an extra minute of high-intensity intervals to their cardiovascular training.

If you're at a gym, make sure to spend a few minutes getting used to the movement of the machine before starting your first "sprint" and a few more minutes cooling down at the end. If you spend 4 weeks in Phase 2, doing the workout twice per week, you'll be up to 13 minutes of HIIT training by the eighth workout.

Phase 2: Building Muscle (Hypertrophy)

Start with a 5- to 10-minute, whole-body warm-up (page 96) and finish with foam rolling and stretching (page 104).

EXERCISE	REPS	SETS	REST
1a. *Beginner:* Dumbbell Squat p. 47 *Intermediate/Advanced:* Barbell Back Squat p. 52 *TRX Option:* TRX Squat p. 51	10–12	2–3	15–30 seconds
1b. *Beginner:* Straight-Leg Dumbbell Dead Lift p. 68 *Intermediate/Advanced:* Straight-Leg Barbell Dead Lift p. 68	10–12	2–3	15–30 seconds
2a. *Beginner:* Back Lunge p. 57 *Intermediate/Advanced:* Back Lunge Off Step p. 58	10–12 each side	2–3	15–30 seconds
2b. *Beginner:* Weighted Glute Bridge p. 72 *Intermediate:* Head-Elevated Hip Thrust p. 73 *Advanced:* Weighted Head-Elevated Hip Thrust p. 73	10–12	2–3	15–30 seconds
3a. *Beginner:* Step-Up p. 79 *Intermediate:* Step-Up with Dumbbells p. 79 *Advanced:* Step-Up with Barbell p. 79	10–12 each side	2–3	15–30 seconds
3b. *Beginner:* Lying Hip Extension p. 81 *Intermediate:* Hip Extension p. 82 *Intermediate/Advanced:* Weighted Hip Extension p. 82	10–12	2–3	15–30 seconds

Optional HIIT for 10 minutes plus 1 additional minute every 2nd workout
    Beginner: 30 seconds work / 90 seconds recovery
    Intermediate/Advanced: 30 seconds work / 60–30 seconds recovery			

Phase 3: Leaning and Cutting

Phase 3 introduces two major changes to the format of the workouts. Rather than perform a single workout for the entire 4 weeks of the phase, we'll be alternating between two different workouts. Perform Workout A on the first legs and glutes training day of the week and Workout B on the second. And instead of performing all exercises as supersets, we'll be starting each workout with straight sets of a single, compound lift.

In Phase 3, you'll be performing 6 to 8 repetitions of each exercise for 2 to 3 (Beginner) or 3 to 4 (Intermediate and Advanced) sets. Always make sure to choose a weight or exercise progression that will nearly fatigue your muscles by the end of the repetition range. You should be lifting heavier in Phase 3 than you were in Phase 2.

Each workout will begin with a single compound lift. You'll perform all reps and sets of this exercise (with the prescribed rest time between sets) before moving on to the isolation supersets.

As in Phases 1 and 2, before beginning the workout, go through the warm-up described in Part 4 of this book. In addition, perform one light or "warm-up" set of the first exercise in the workout; for example, in Workout A, you'll do 6 to 8 Bulgarian Split Squats on each leg with a light weight or body weight only at the end of your usual warm-up. Note that this warm-up set does not count toward the set total for this exercise.

The workout finishes with a Tabata interval, cool-down, foam rolling, and stretching.

Up until now, you've been using a 2-0-2-0 tempo on your lifts; counting to 2 on each of the concentric (2) and eccentric (2) phases of your lifts, with little to no pause at the top (0) or bottom (0). During Phase 3, Intermediate and Advanced lifters might consider increasing the speed of the concentric phase of their lifts, thereby adopting a 1-0-2-0 or even a 1-0-3-0 tempo. Changing the tempo of your lifts has a similar effect to changing the load and the repetition range; it shocks your muscles and often results in improved strength gains and muscle growth. Note that you don't need to use the same tempo with every exercise. Never compromise your form just to increase the speed of a concentric contraction.

Aim to progress one exercise each and every time you perform the workout, either by increasing your weights or choosing a more challenging exercise from the options given. Remember that your repetition number is likely to drop to the lower end of the suggested rep range when you first progress an exercise.

Do this workout twice per week, with 48 to 72 hours between sessions. If you have the time and energy AND if you're feeling like you're not losing fat at the rate you'd like to be, you may add an extra HIIT workout, if you'd like, on a day when you're not training your legs. Continue with the HIIT training protocol outlined in Phase 2, adding 1 minute to your total training time each week.

Again, feel free to extend Phase 3 of the program for another week or two. Then take a well-earned week away from the gym!

Phase 3: Leaning and Cutting Workout A

Start with a 5- to 10-minute, whole-body warm-up (page 96) and finish with foam rolling and stretching (page 104).

EXERCISE	REPS	SETS	REST
1. *Beginner:* Bulgarian Split Squat p. 53 *Intermediate:* Dumbbell Bulgarian Split Squat p. 53 *Advanced:* Braced Bulgarian Split Squat p. 53 *TRX Option:* TRX Bulgarian Split Squat p. 54	6–8 each side	2–4	60–90 seconds
2a. *Beginner:* Dumbbell Lateral Lunge p. 61 *Intermediate/Advanced:* Alternating Dumbbell Lateral Lunge p. 61	6–8 each side	2–4	15–30 seconds
2b. *Beginner:* Head-Elevated Hip Thrust p. 73 *Intermediate/Advanced:* Weighted Head-Elevated Hip Thrust p. 73	6–8	2–4	15–30 seconds
3a. *Beginner/Intermediate:* Weighted Lying Leg Raise p. 84 *Intermediate/Advanced:* Standing Cable Hip Abduction p. 85	6–8 each side	2–4	15–30 seconds
3b. *Beginner:* Single-Leg Hamstring Curl on the Ball p. 64 *Intermediate/Advanced:* Single-Leg Hamstring Curl on the Ball with Hip Extension p. 64 *TRX Option:* TRX Hamstring Curl p. 65	6–8 each side	2–4	15–30 seconds
Tabata: 20 seconds work / 10 seconds recovery x 8 cycles; choose one of the following: Burpee p. 88, Squat Jumps p. 90, or Split Squat Jumps p. 91			

Phase 3: Leaning and Cutting Workout B

Start with a 5- to 10-minute, whole-body warm-up (page 96) and finish with foam rolling and stretching (page 104).

EXERCISE	REPS	SETS	REST
1. *Beginner:* Single-Leg Bent-Knee Dead Lift p. 69 *Intermediate/Advanced:* Single-Leg Straight-Leg Dead Lift p. 70	6–8 each side	2–4	60–90 seconds
2a. *Beginner:* Barbell Stationary Lunge p. 56 *Intermediate/Advanced:* Barbell Walking Lunge p. 59	6–8 each side	2–4	15–30 seconds
2b. *Beginner:* Double-Arm Hip Swing p. 75 *Intermediate/Advanced:* Single-Arm Hip Swing p. 75	6–8 each side	2–4	15–30 seconds
3a. *Beginner:* Goblet Squat p. 48 *Intermediate:* Dumbbell Front Squat p. 49 *Advanced:* Barbell Front Squat p. 50	6–8	2–4	15–30 seconds
3b. *Beginner:* Forearm Plank with Hip Abduction p. 86 *Intermediate/Advanced:* Forearm Plank with Weighted Hip Abduction p. 87	30 seconds each side	2–4	15–30 seconds
Tabata: 20 seconds work / 10 seconds recovery x 8 cycles; choose one of the following: Speed Skaters p. 92, Two-Foot Lateral Hops p. 93, or Side Shuffles p. 93			

You've Finished the Program: Now What?

Congratulations! You've finished the 12-week *Ultimate Booty Workouts* program. If you followed the principles of consistency and progression we discussed earlier, and made the appropriate changes to your diet, you should be noticing a higher, firmer, rounder, and more sculpted derriere. But don't stop now. In all likelihood, there's still room for improvement and at the very least, you'll want to maintain the gains you've made over the past 3 months.

There are a couple of different directions you could take with your training, depending on your fitness goals.

Looking to continue focusing on glute and leg training? Take a week off (rest is good for you) and then repeat the entire 12 weeks of the program, but with heavier weights (and more challenging versions of the exercises) the second time around. If you started the program as a Beginner, try the Intermediate exercise options. As you go back to Phase 1, you'll find that the weights that challenged you the first time through will no longer be enough to generate muscular fatigue. You can continue cycling through the three phases of this program as many times as you like; this technique of varying the loads and repetitions is called "periodization" and is practiced widely in the strength-training community. Just make sure to take a "rest" or "de-loading" week every time you finish Phase 3.

Wanting to train other body parts as well, but not lose the lower body gains you've worked so hard for? Cut your targeted leg and glutes training days back to once a week and repeat the Phases 2 and 3 of the program. Add in 2 to 3 days of whole body, metabolic strength training, working all muscle groups in a single session, focusing on compound, bang-for-your-buck exercises. Depending on your age and experience, you may need to continue with twice-a-week legs and glutes training to avoid deconditioning. Continue recording your workouts in your journal to determine the best training schedule for your body.

Still feeling the need to reduce body fat? Extend Phase 3 by another month and add an additional cardio interval workout on your "rest" days. As mentioned previously, HIIT-style training will be far more beneficial to your fat loss goals than endurance training. Work harder, not longer.

Regardless of which option you decide on, make sure you're challenging yourself by regularly progressing the exercises and loads. As a general rule of thumb, aim to switch up your training every 4 to 6 weeks, before your body adapts to the stimulus and stops responding to your workouts.

PART 3
THE EXERCISES

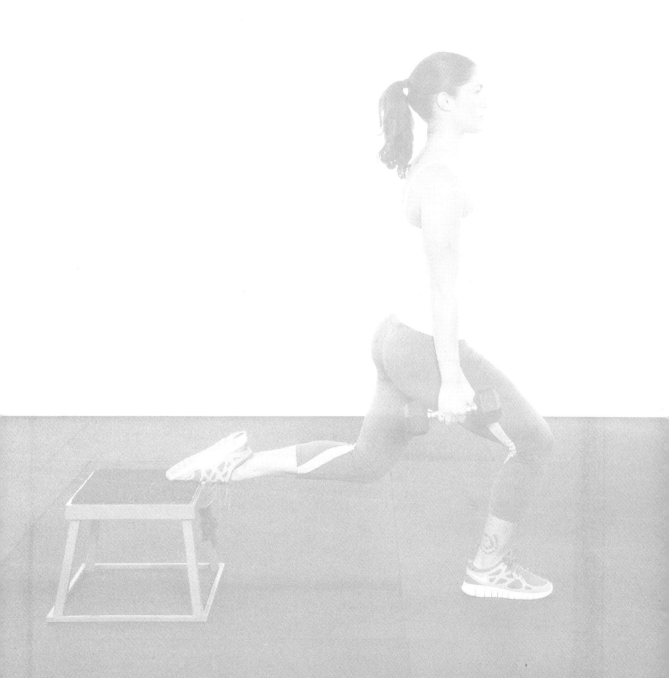

Squats

Perfecting your squat form is key to developing strong, muscular glutes. In Phase 1, if you've never squatted before or you find it difficult to get much depth on your Bodyweight Squats, try starting with the Ball Squat. Once you've developed some leg and glute strength, progress to Bodyweight Squats before adding dumbbells to the movement. Plié and Goblet Squat variations not only increase the focus on the glutes, they also recruit the muscles of the inner thighs. And who doesn't want strong inner thighs?

In Phase 2, we'll be progressing your squats by adding load and moving that load up and away from your feet. Beginners should continue with the Dumbbell Squat, holding weights either beside your body at arm's length or up at shoulder height. Intermediate and Advanced lifters may move on to Barbell Back Squats, aiming to keep shoulders back and down, neck neutral, eyes forward, and working through as big a range of motion as possible.

Back Squats can be performed with a standard barbell or an Olympic bar. Note that the Olympic bar weighs 45 pounds without plates, and due to its length may feel heavier and more unwieldy than a standard barbell of the same weight. I always start clients with a standard barbell and move them "up" to the Olympic bar when they can no longer press the weight of the barbell up and over their head to get it into Back Squat position. For more details on squatting with an O-bar, see page 28.

In order to increase the work on the glutes and quads, during Phase 3 we'll be (1) moving the weight away from the ground and out in front of your body and (2) incorporating the more challenging split stance.

You may find that holding dumbbells or a barbell in front of your shoulders reduces the depth of your squat. That's okay. Concentrate on maintaining good form and slowly increasing your squat depth as your glutes and lower back get stronger.

Beginners will perform the Goblet Squat at this point. Intermediate and Advanced lifters will progress through Dumbbell and Barbell Front Squats. Feel free to use an Olympic Bar for this exercise when a 45 pound dumbbell is no longer enough to fatigue your muscles by the end of the set.

Single-Leg (or pistol) Squats are the king of glute and leg exercises, requiring strength, power, balance, and a great kinesthetic sense. But chances are, unless you've been doing lower body training for a considerable length of time, you won't yet have the strength to support yourself on just one leg through a full range-of-motion squat.

Enter the Bulgarian Split Squat. Part lunge, part single-leg squat, it's an exercise that never seems to get any easier, no matter how long you practice it. Concentrate on the muscles of the supporting leg, resisting the temptation to let the trailing leg help you return to standing.

BALL SQUAT

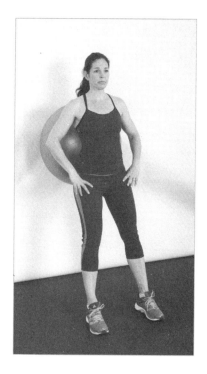 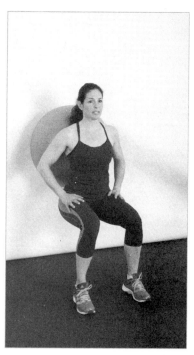

1 Standing with your back to a wall, place a stability ball between your lower back and the wall. Walk feet out in front of you, placing them a bit wider than hip-distance apart, with toes pointing forward or turned out slightly.

2 Pulling your shoulder blades back and down, lower your torso toward the floor by bending your knees and rolling the ball up your back. Stop when your thighs are parallel to the ground, making sure that your knees are not extended beyond your toes and that your chest and shoulders are still facing forward. If you can't see your toes, walk your feet farther from the wall.

Squeeze your glutes together and push through your heels to return to standing.

PLIÉ BALL SQUAT

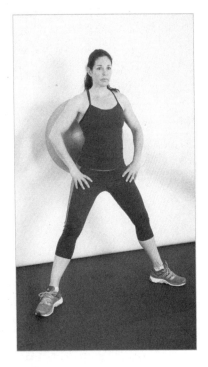
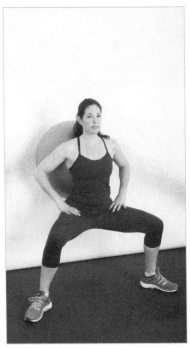

1 Starting in the same position as described for the Ball Squat, step your feet farther apart and turn your toes out, like a ballerina.

2 Keeping your shoulders back and down, lower your torso and butt toward the floor, allowing your knees to fall out over your toes.

Squeeze your glutes and draw your inner thighs toward one another while you push through your heels to return to standing.

VARIATION: Intermediate lifters may increase the difficulty of this movement by holding a pair of dumbbells either down at their sides or at shoulder height.

BODYWEIGHT SQUAT

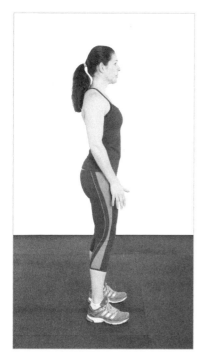

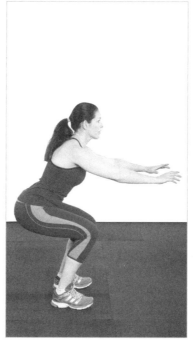

DUMBBELL VARIATION:
Follow the above instructions for a Bodyweight Squat while holding a pair of dumbbells at your sides. More advanced lifters may choose to hold their weights at shoulder height; the higher the load is held, the greater the effort required to return to standing at the end of the squat.

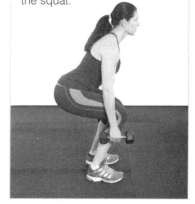

1 Start by standing with your feet a bit wider than hip-width apart, toes pointing forward or slightly turned out, belly button pulled in toward your spine and shoulders back and down.

2 Hold your arms out in front of your body, and lower your rear end toward the floor by hinging at the hip and bending your knees and ankles. Maintain a forward gaze, with your chest open, weight in your heels, and knees behind your toes.

Squeeze your glute cheeks and push through your heels to return to standing. Arms can either remain out in front or swung down to your sides on the up phase of the movement.

GOBLET SQUAT

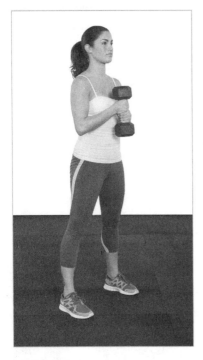
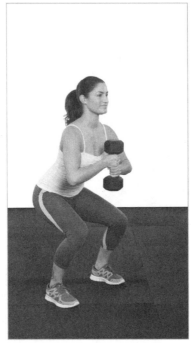

1 Stand with your feet significantly wider than hip-distance apart (toes may either face forward or be turned out slightly) and hold a single, heavy dumbbell at chest height. The weight should be braced against your body with elbows tucked in.

2 Lower your butt toward the floor, keeping your shoulders back and down and chest facing forward, until your elbows touch the insides of your thighs.

Contract glutes and push through heels to return to standing.

DUMBBELL FRONT SQUAT

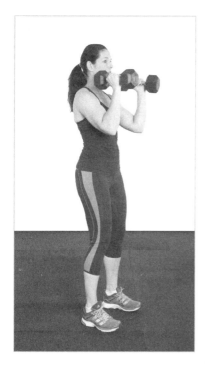 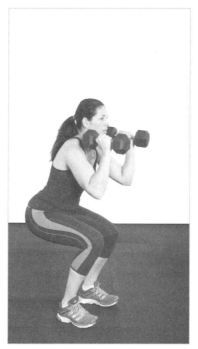

1 Stand with feet your under your hips (or slightly wider if that's more comfortable for you), and hold a pair of dumbbells just in front of your shoulders. At no point during the exercise should the weights be resting on your body.

2 Sit back into the squat by hinging at the hip and bending at the knees and ankles. Concentrate on pushing your butt back while keeping your eyes and chest facing forward. Knees should remain behind the toes throughout.

Squeeze your glute cheeks and push through your heels to return to standing.

Complete all reps with minimal rest between. The farther down you squat, the more work required to return to standing.

BARBELL FRONT SQUAT

Proper form is ABSOLUTELY NECESSARY with this movement to avoid injury. Start with a light barbell and add load only when you've mastered the exercise. For more details on the safe use of an Olympic bar, see page 28.

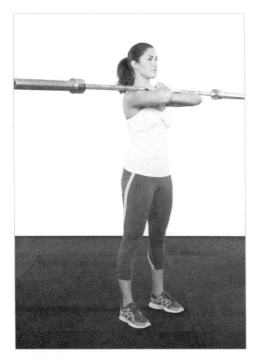 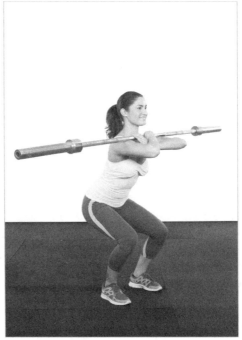

1 Begin by standing with your feet slightly wider than your hips, toes facing forward or slightly turned out. Place a barbell across your biceps, crossing your arms to hold it securely in place. Lift your upper arms until they're parallel to the floor. Elbows will be at shoulder level and facing forward to keep the bar from rolling off.

2 Hinge at the hips, knees, and ankles to sit back into the squat. Keep your arms up, eyes forward, and torso tall.

Squeeze your abs and glutes, and push through heels to return to standing. Repeat all repetitions with minimal rest between

TRX SQUAT

You can improve the depth of your squat using the TRX.

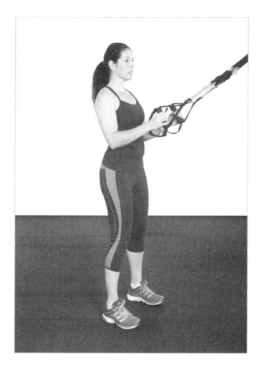
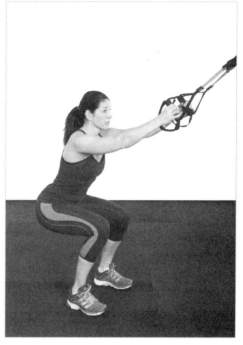

1 Adjust the length of the TRX straps until the handles are hanging about 3 feet from the floor. Holding the handles lightly, stand with your feet slightly wider than hip-distance apart.

2 Drop your rear back and down toward the floor, hinging at the hip and leaning forward slightly to counterbalance your backside.

Push through heels to return to standing, using the TRX for support.

Ensure that your legs are doing most of the work; this is not an upper body exercise.

BARBELL BACK SQUAT

For more details on the safe use of an Olympic bar, see page 28.

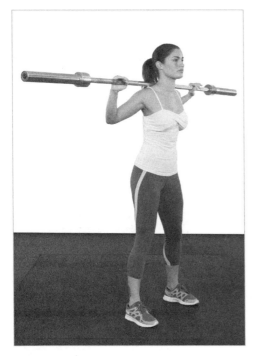 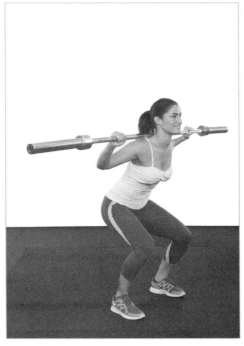

1 Standing with your feet approximately hip-width apart, grasp a barbell in both hands using an overhand grip. Bend your knees slightly, tighten your core, and push through your heels to raise the bar up and overhead, guiding it to gently rest behind your head, across your shoulder blades. The bar should NEVER rest on your neck; draw your shoulder blades down and back to create a "ledge" for it to sit on. Doing so will also allow you to maintain an upright, forward-looking posture throughout the move.

2 Sit back into the squat, sinking as low as you can by bending at the hips, knees, and ankles.

Push through your heels to return to the starting position.

When all reps are completed, press bar up and over your head before placing it on the ground.

BULGARIAN SPLIT SQUAT

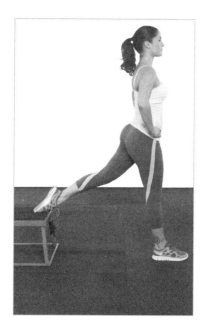

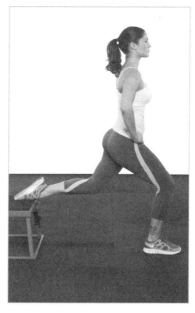

1 Begin by standing with your back toward a low step or weight bench. Reach back with your left leg and place your foot on the bench, shoelaces down. Hop your right leg forward, so that when you lower the left knee toward the floor, your right knee isn't shooting out over your toes. Hands can be held down at your sides, across your chest (more challenging), or behind your head (even more challenging). Avoid leaning forward; you want to maintain an upright posture, with eyes focused on the horizon throughout the movement.

2 Start your set by contracting your abs, pulling your shoulders back and down, and lowering your back knee toward the floor.

Pause at the bottom, then tighten your glutes and push through the foot on the floor to return to standing.

Complete all repetitions on one side, then switch to the other side and repeat.

DUMBBELL VARIATION:
Intermediate and Advanced lifters may make this exercise more challenging by adding load. Hold a pair of dumbbells at your sides while following the above instructions.

BRACED VARIATION:
Advanced lifters can increase the difficulty of the move and add a core challenge by holding a single, heavy weight plate out in front of you while you execute the movement. The farther the weight is held from your body, the more difficult the exercise. Make sure you keep your shoulders down and away from your ears and your abs engaged to support the muscles of your mid and lower back.

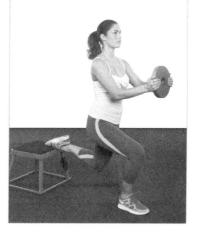

TRX BULGARIAN SPLIT SQUAT

The higher the straps are from the floor, the more challenging the exercise.

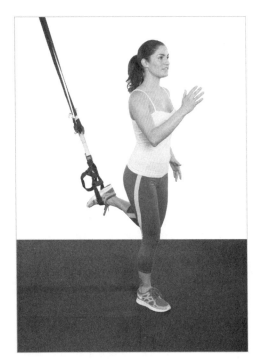
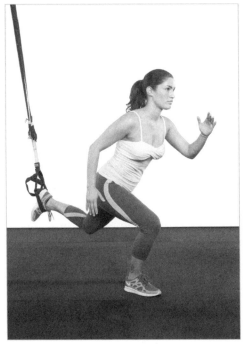

1 Starting with straps butterflied to create a single loop approximately 18 inches from the floor, stand facing away from the TRX and reach back with one leg to place your foot through the loop.

2 Making sure that your stance is wide enough to prevent the front knee from shooting out over the toe, start your set by contracting your abs, pulling your shoulders back and down, and lowering your back knee toward the floor.

Pause at the bottom, then tighten your glutes and push through the foot on the floor to return to standing.

Complete all repetitions on one side, then switch to the other side and repeat.

Lunges

No legs and glutes workout would be complete without lunges. Because lunges are performed on one side of the body at a time, they not only help to reduce left-right muscular inequalities, they also challenge your balance, thereby requiring increased core activation. Make sure you spend time perfecting your bodyweight Stationary Lunges before adding load to the movement and advancing to Back Lunges. When people new to lower body exercise complain about sore knees, poor lunge form is almost always the culprit.

Lateral Band Walks and Dumbbell Lateral Lunges are a great way to target the medial glutes. Make sure that toes stay pointing forward throughout these side–to–side exercises; outward pointing toes are a sure sign that your stronger, more powerful quadriceps are running the show.

In Phase 2, we'll progress our Back Lunges by (1) performing all repetitions on one side (beginning with the nondominant side) before switching to the other and (2) lunging backward off a low step. Beginner, Intermediate, and Advanced exercisers will all add load to their lunges, either by holding dumbbells at their sides or by placing a barbell across the back of their shoulders (see Barbell Back Squat for details on barbell placement).

As mentioned earlier, working the muscles of the lower body in more than one plane of motion is essential to building a strong and sculpted behind. Lateral Lunges strengthen the gluteus medius as well as the muscles of the inner thigh. Beginners will perform all repetitions on one side before moving to the other. Intermediate and Advanced lifters will alternate sides, a more challenging move because proper foot placement must be reattained with every repetition.

In Phase 3 we'll progress our lunges by increasing the distance between the added load and the ground; the farther the weights are from our feet, the more work the quads and glutes have to do. Both Beginners and Intermediate/Advanced exercisers will use a barbell for this movement. See instructions for safely placing the barbell across your shoulders in the description of the Barbell Back Squat (page 52).

STATIONARY LUNGE

Beginners will want to perfect this movement with body weight alone. Intermediate lifters can hold a dumbbell in each hand to increase the load.

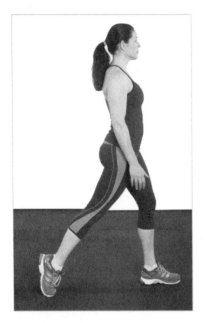

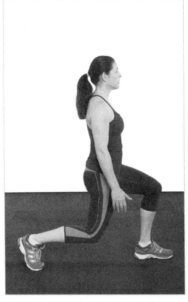

BARBELL VARIATION:
Perform a Stationary Lunge, but with a barbell held across the back of your shoulders. Make sure your hands are placed well beyond shoulder-width apart and that the bar rests on your shoulder blades rather than your neck.

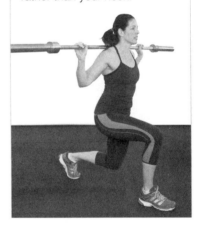

1 Begin by standing with feet hip-distance apart. Take a large step back with your right foot, maintaining the distance between feet, and lift your right heel off the floor so that you're balancing on your toes or the ball of your foot.

2 Keeping your upper body tall and left knee behind the toes of your left foot, drop your right knee down toward the floor. Aim for 90-degree angles at both knee joints. If you have limited range of motion in your knees due to tightness or injury, drop only as low as you comfortably can.

Squeeze your glutes and push through the LEFT heel to return to standing. Avoid pushing off with the back toes to maximize gluteal involvement.

Complete all repetitions on the right side then repeat with the other leg.

BACK LUNGE

Maintain a slow and steady tempo and avoid rushing; rushing tends to lead to improper back foot placement and hyperflexion of the front knee over the front foot. Practice this exercise without weights before attempting it with dumbbells.

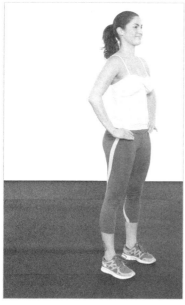

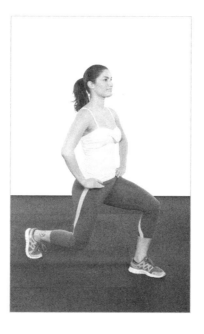

> **VARIATION:** More advanced exercisers may progress the exercise by alternating legs until all repetitions have been completed on each side.

1 Begin by standing with feet hip-distance apart.

2 Take a large step back with your right foot, maintaining the distance between feet, and lift your right heel off the floor so that you're balancing on your toes or the ball of your foot.

Return to standing by contracting left glute and pushing through the left heel.

Perform all repetitions on one side before switching to the other.

BACK LUNGE OFF STEP

This exercise can be progressed by increasing the height of the step as well as the weight of the dumbbells or barbell.

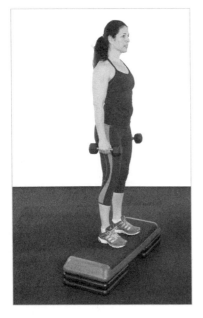 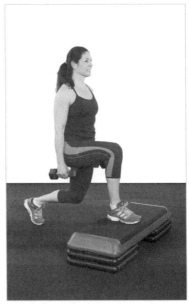

1 Start by standing on a low step, with a dumbbell in each hand or a barbell across the back of your shoulders.

2 Step back and off the step with your left leg, immediately dropping your left knee down into the lunge position. The back heel will be off the ground and torso will be perpendicular to the floor. Knees should be bent at approximately 90 degrees and your front knee should remain behind the front toes.

Engage your glutes and press through your right heel (the foot on the step) to rise and return your right leg to the step.

Complete all reps on the right side before switching to the left.

BARBELL WALKING LUNGE

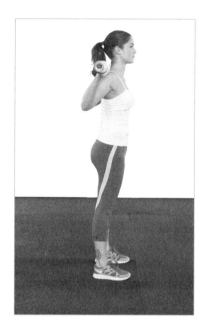 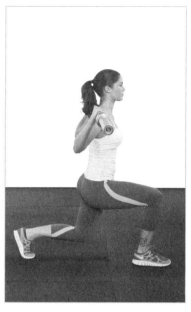 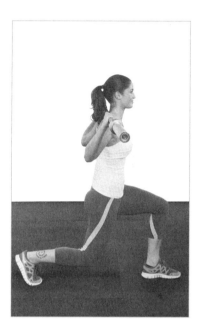

1 Begin by standing with your feet hip-distance apart and a barbell held across the back of your shoulders with your hands placed well beyond shoulder-width apart.

2 Keeping your eyes looking forward and torso tall, take a step forward with the right foot, lowering the left knee toward the floor and ending up in a position where both your front and back knees form 90-degree angles; avoid letting your front knee drift out beyond your toes.

3 Pushing through your right (front) heel, return to standing and step forward with your left (back) foot, dropping immediately back down into the lunge position.

Continue alternating legs, walking forward until all repetitions have been completed on each side.

LATERAL BAND WALK

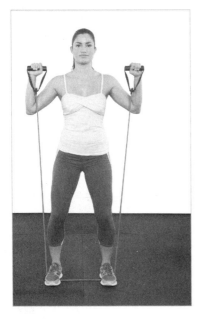 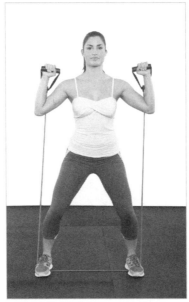 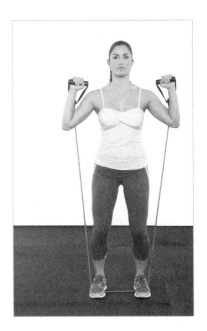

1 Stand on a resistance band with your feet hip-distance apart and the handles of the band held either at your waist or behind your shoulders (depending on your height, your strength, and the length of your band, you may or may not be able to hold the band at shoulder height).

2 Pulling your shoulders back and down and bending slightly at the knees, take a step to the left, pushing against the resistance of the band with the outside of your hip, leg, and foot.

3 Step your right foot in toward the left and repeat until you've completed all repetitions on the left leg. Make sure that the toes of both feet continue to point forward throughout the entire set to prevent the quadriceps from taking over.

Switch sides and repeat. Note that when practicing the Lateral Band Walk during the warm-up, you'll be alternating sides every second repetition rather than performing a long set of reps on one side at a time.

DUMBBELL LATERAL LUNGE

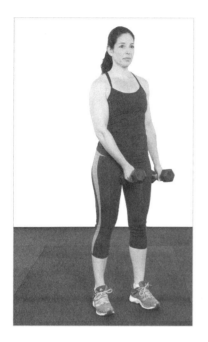

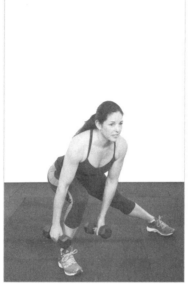

ALTERNATING VARIATION:
Do the Lateral Lunge by alternating sides until all repetitions have been completed on both sides.

1 Stand with your feet hip-distance apart and hold a dumbbell in each hand in front of your quads.

2 Step the right leg out wide to the side. Keeping the toes of both feet pointing forward, bend at the hip, push your glutes down, and lower your chest toward the right thigh. At the bottom of the movement, your right leg will be bent, your left leg will be straight, and your back will be flat and almost parallel to the floor.

Touch the dumbbells to the floor on either side of your right foot.

Using your inner and outer thighs, pull yourself back up to the starting position.

Complete all repetitions on the right side before switching sides.

Hamstring Curls

"Hip hinge" exercises are used primarily for building hamstring strength and emphasizing the "hamstring-glute tie-in," which is important both for lifting the butt and for balancing the stronger, front-of-the-body quadriceps. Although they may look easy, Hamstring Curls on the Ball are an intense isolation exercise, requiring balance, core strength, and hamstring endurance. Even the Intermediate and Advanced lifters in my gym practice them regularly.

HAMSTRING CURL ON THE BALL

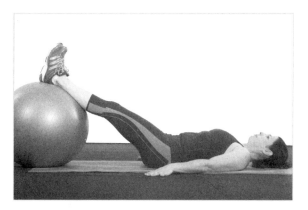

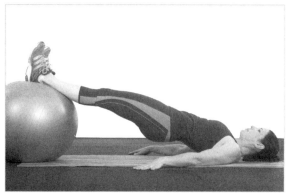

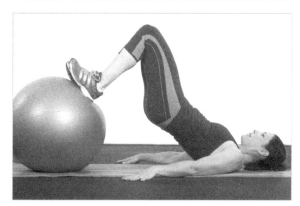

1 Lay face up (supine) on a mat with both feet on top of an exercise ball. Extend your arms out to your sides at shoulder height (not shown) and press your palms into the floor.

2 Tighten your glutes and core to lift your midsection up and off the mat. Your body should be in a straight line from your shoulders (on the floor) to your heels (on the ball).

3 Keeping your hips up and off the mat, bend both knees and use your heels to roll the ball in toward your rear end. Straighten your legs and push the ball away to finish the move. Make sure that you keep your hips high and butt off the mat until you've finished the set.

To increase the balance challenge of the exercise, move your arms down to the sides of your body (as pictured here). Even more challenging? Take your hands off the floor and extend both arms toward the ceiling, directly over your chest.

SINGLE-LEG HAMSTRING CURL ON THE BALL

Building on the two-legged Hamstring Curls we practiced in Phase 1, Phase 3 progresses the exercise to work hamstrings one at a time. Beginners will perform the basic curl, Intermediate and Advanced exercisers will add a hip extension to the top of the movement.

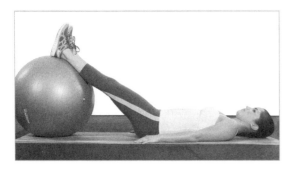

1 Lay face up (supine) on a mat with both feet on top of an exercise ball. Place your arms at your sides and press your palms into the floor.

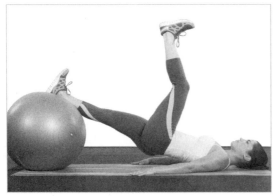

2 Engaging your abs and glutes, lift hips up and off the mat and extend the left leg up toward the ceiling.

3 Using the right leg only, curl the ball in toward your butt, keeping your left leg in the air and hips up and off the mat until all repetitions are complete.

Switch legs and repeat.

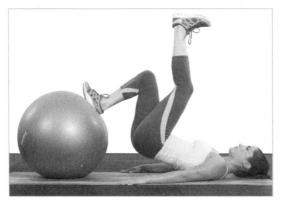

VARIATION WITH HIP EXTENSION: Perform the Single-Leg Hamstring Curl as described above, but as you pull the ball in, squeeze your glutes and lift your hips up, so that the thigh of the leg you're curling the ball with forms a straight line with your torso at the top of the movement. Lower hips as you roll the ball back out to the starting position. Complete all repetitions on one leg before switching legs and repeating.

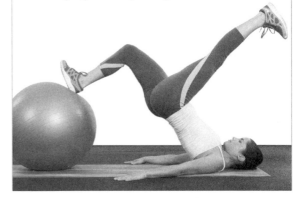

TRX HAMSTRING CURL

This can be done with or without hip extension. Note that this movement reverts to working both legs at the same time.

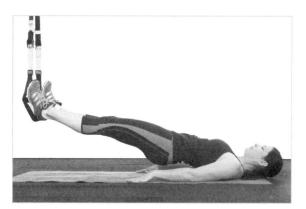

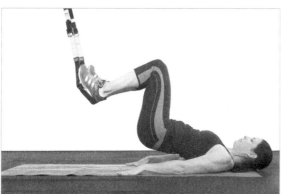

1 Starting with straps even and approximately 18 inches off the ground, lay on your back and place your heels in the loops of the TRX. Although it may feel as if your feet aren't secure, once you lift your hips up and off the ground, the weight of your legs will ensure that your feet don't slip out of the straps.

2 Arms can either be placed on the ground at shoulder level or alongside your body, the second option being more challenging than the first. Keeping even pressure on both handles, pull heels in towards your bottom.

Pause and slowly return to starting position, making sure not to lower your butt to the ground between repetitions.

Adding a hip extension to the end of the move (as described on page 64) is optional and extremely challenging!

Dead Lifts

When first introduced to Dead Lifts, many exercisers have difficulty distinguishing them from a squat. While the beginning of the movement may appear similar, Dead Lifts require a "pull" rather than a "push" to return to standing. Make sure you're focusing on the hamstrings and lower back to complete the lift, not the quads.

During Phase 2, we'll be progressing our hip hinges by performing dead lifts with straightened legs. Doing so reduces the involvement of the quadriceps and encourages the hamstrings and glutes to do more of the work. Note that even in the straight-leg position, there should always be a slight bend at the knees. Never lock your knees

when lifting. You'll also feel your lower back, particularly if it's the weakest link in your core. Focus on keeping the back straight and reaching only as far down as is comfortable (or perhaps just a bit uncomfortable...). Gradually increase your depth and range of motion as the muscles of your backside get stronger.

As with the Bulgarian Split Squat (page 53), Phase 3's Dead Lifts will also be executed on one leg. In addition to building your hamstrings and glutes, Single-Leg Dead Lifts will also improve your balance and strengthen your deep core stabilizers.

Take your time with this exercise. Plant your supporting foot firmly on the floor and find a

stationary point in the distance to focus on. If absolutely necessary, you may use a chair or the wall for support, but your eventual goal should be to perform the exercise without assistance.

Beginners will start with the bent-knee version of the exercise, as it places less stress on the muscles of the lower back and helps to safely teach the pulling motion required to return to standing. Intermediate and Advanced exercisers may progress to the straight-leg version, provided they feel no pain or stress on the lumbar spine when doing so.

BENT-LEG DUMBBELL DEAD LIFT

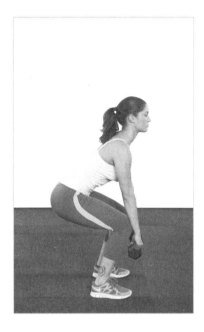 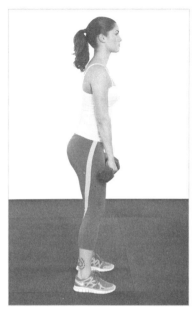

1 Stand with your feet hip distance (or slightly wider) apart and hold a pair of dumbbells directly in front of your thighs, knuckles facing away from your body.

Bend your knees slightly, hinge forward at the hip, and reach your butt back as you lower your weights toward the floor.

2 Pull yourself back up to standing using your hamstrings, glutes, and lower back. Think about "shaving your legs" with your weights and maintaining a straight back throughout the exercise.

When you reach the top of the movement, push your hips forward and pull your shoulders back and down. Exaggerating the finish will ensure that you've activated the correct muscles and performed the exercise through its entire range of motion.

STRAIGHT-LEG DUMBBELL DEAD LIFT

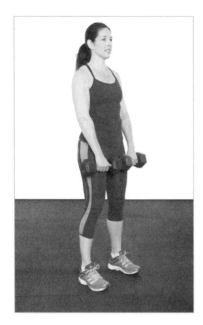

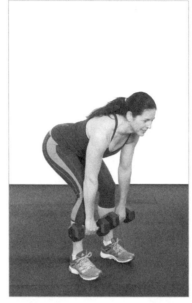

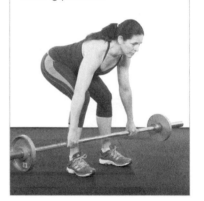

BARBELL VARIATION:
Replace the dumbbells with a barbell and follow the instructions for the Straight-Leg Dumbbell Dead Lift. Remember to hold the barbell with a wide, forward facing grip and to "shave your legs" with the bar when returning to the starting position.

1 Stand with your feet hip distance (or slightly wider) apart and hold a pair of dumbbells directly in front of your thighs, knuckles facing away from your body. Despite the name of the exercise, you will maintain a slight bend in the knees throughout.

2 With your shoulders pulled back and down and hinging ONLY at the hip, slowly lower the weights toward the floor.

Tightening your core and gluteals, pull yourself back to standing using your hamstrings, glutes, and lower back. At the top of the movement, push your hips forward slightly and press your shoulders back and down.

SINGLE-LEG BENT-KNEE DEAD LIFT

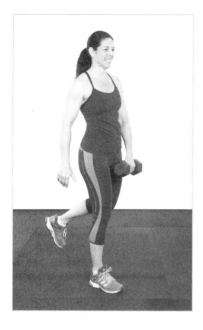 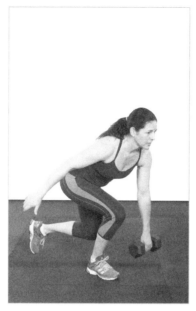

1 Start by standing on your right foot, maintaining a soft bend in the knee and lifting your left leg up and off the ground, slightly behind your body. Your torso should be tall with shoulders back and down.

2 Holding a heavy dumbbell in the left hand, hinge your hips slightly, reaching your butt back as you bend the right knee and reach the weight down toward your right foot. Maintain a straight back, with chest facing forward and eye focus about 3 yards in front of your foot.

Simultaneously push through your right heel and pull with your hamstrings and lower back to return to standing, exaggerating the end of the movement by pushing your hips forward and shoulders back.

Perform all reps on the right before switching to the other side and repeating.

SINGLE-LEG STRAIGHT-LEG DEAD LIFT

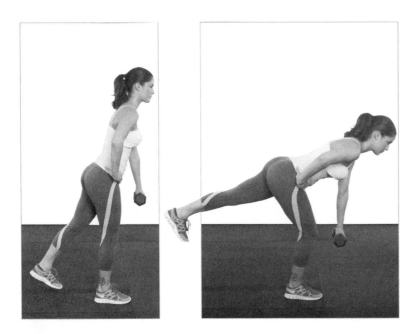

1 Start by standing on your right foot, maintaining a soft bend in the knee and lifting your left leg up and off the ground, slightly behind your body. Despite the name of the exercise, you will maintain a small bend in the supporting leg throughout.

2 Holding a dumbbell in your left hand, hinge forward at the hips, without increasing the bend at the knee, and reach the weight down toward your right foot. As you hinge, raise your straight left leg up until it's nearly parallel to the floor; it will act as a counterbalance to any forward momentum and keep you from tipping over.

Pull with your hamstrings and lower back to return to standing, exaggerating the end of the movement by pushing your hips forward and shoulders back.

Perform all reps on the right before switching sides.

Glute Bridges

Bridging is one of the best exercises for learning to "fire up" or "turn on" your glutes. Not only will glute bridges help to build and define your butt, they'll also strengthen your abs and lower back. Begin with the Basic Glute Bridge, making sure that glutes and core remain tight and engaged for the entire set. Increase the difficulty of the exercise first with the Feet-Elevated Glute Bridge and then with the Weighted Glute Bridge.

In Phase 2, we'll increase the difficulty of our glute bridges by adding weight (Beginner) and elevating our heads and shoulders (Intermediate and Advanced). The greater the elevation of the upper body, the more challenging the exercise.

In Phase 3, we'll continue to progress our Hip Thrusts by both elevating the head (Beginners) and adding weight to the Head-Elevated Hip Thrust (Intermediate and Advanced). Weight options include SandBells, dumbbells, weight plates, and even barbells. Always use your hands to support the weight and keep it from rolling off your hips.

BASIC GLUTE BRIDGE

To increase the effectiveness of the exercise, don't rest your butt on the floor between reps; remember that increasing the time a muscle remains under tension leads to faster strength gains and better muscular endurance.

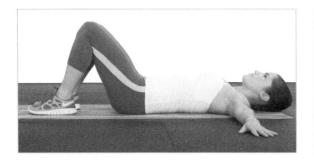

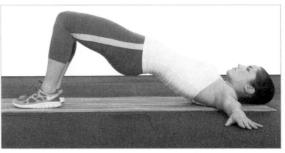

1 Lay down on the floor or a mat, face up, with feet on the floor directly below your bent knees. Extend arms out to your sides at shoulder level.

2 Contracting the muscles of your belly and backside, push your hips up toward the ceiling so that only your feet, shoulders, and arms remain in contact with the floor.

Slowly lower your hips toward the floor, keeping your back straight and abdominals engaged.

Perform all repetitions before allowing your glutes to return to the floor.

FEET-ELEVATED VARIATION: Perform exactly like the Basic Glute Bridge, but with feet elevated on either a plyo box, step, BOSU, or weight bench. The higher the feet are placed, the more

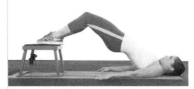

challenging the exercise; start with an elevation of 4 to 6 inches and progress to an 18-inch weight bench over time. Choosing an unstable surface (like a BOSU) to rest your feet on will provide an additional balance challenge and further engage your core stabilization muscles.

WEIGHTED VARIATION: Increase the difficulty of both the Basic Glute Bridge and the Feet-Elevated Glute Bridge by performing the exercise with a weight placed across your hips. Try

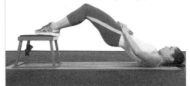

adding a weight plate or a SandBell; both are flat and will stay securely in place as you execute your reps. A dumbbell or barbell can also be used, but you may need to hold it lightly to ensure it doesn't roll or fall off.

HEAD-ELEVATED HIP THRUST

This exercise can also be done on a low step, BOSU, or weight bench.

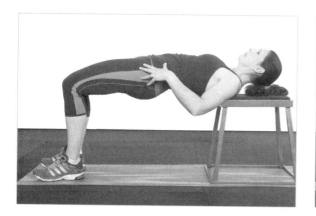

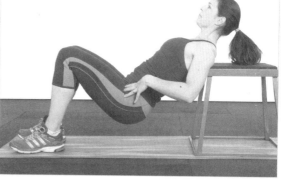

1 Place your head and shoulders on a plyo box. With your feet on the ground and knees directly over the toes, assume a "tabletop" position, with hips high and glutes and core engaged.

2 Lower your buttocks toward the floor before thrusting your hips forcefully up toward the ceiling.

WEIGHTED VARIATION: Begin in the same position as for Head-Elevated Hip Thrust, but with a dumbbell, weight plate, or SandBell placed across your hips. Lower your hips toward the floor, and without pausing at the bottom of the movement, thrust your hips up toward the ceiling, holding on to the weight with your hands to keep it from falling off.

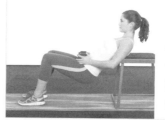

Hip Swings

A standing version of the Hip Thrust, Hip Swings are a great metabolic addition to your Phase 3 workouts. In addition to strengthening your hamstrings, glutes, and core, if you use a heavy-enough weight, you'll also feel your shoulders, biceps, and forearm flexors working. One of the best "whole body" exercises around.

Beginners will start with Double-Arm Hip Swings. Intermediate and Advanced lifters will use one arm at a time, completing all reps on one side before switching to the other. Note that moving from double to single arm swings often requires a decrease in the weight lifted. You can perform this exercise with either a kettlebell or a single heavy dumbbell, depending on the equipment available to you.

Regardless, remember that this exercise is meant primarily as a hip exercise; your arms and core are merely an extension of your hips.

DOUBLE-ARM HIP SWING

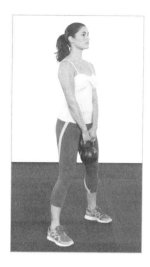 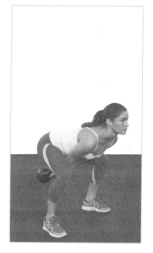 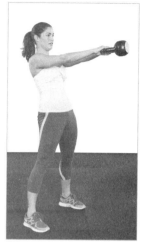 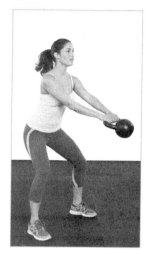

1 Standing with your feet apart, toes turned out slightly, and either a kettlebell or a heavy dumbbell held between two hands, pull your shoulders back and down and engage your abs.

2 Hinge forward slightly from the hips and reach your hands back between your legs; keep your shins approximately perpendicular to the floor throughout the movement.

3 With your arms held long, thrust your hips forward so that weight is propelled upward to about shoulder height.

4 Let gravity return the weight back to its starting position and immediately begin the next rep.

Keep your neck neutral throughout the exercise; tucking it slightly will prevent both neck strain and rounding of the lumbar spine. Swings have a momentum of their own; find your rhythm and maintain this tempo for the entire set. If you can swing the weight up above shoulder height, you need a heavier weight.

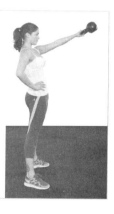

SINGLE-ARM VARIATION: Start in the same position as described above for the Double-Arm Hip Swing, but with one hand holding the kettlebell or weight and the other placed either on your hip or behind your lower back. Perform all repetitions on one side, ensuring that your chest and torso remain facing forward throughout the set, chin slightly tucked to prevent both neck strain and rounding of the back. Switch sides and repeat.

Planks

I know. You thought that planks were just a core exercise. Why then, include them in a workout designed to strengthen and sculpt your derriere?

The truth is, planks are a whole-body exercise. To hold a good-form plank, you not only need to engage your abdominal muscles, you also need to support your upper body with your arms, shoulders, and back and your lower body with quads, glutes, and hamstrings.

Recall that one of the functions of your glutes is to support and protect your lower back. Once you can hold a Forearm Plank on Knees for 45 seconds, progress to the Forearm Plank on Toes. Fire up your glutes the next time you plank and I bet you'll be able to hold it longer and without lower back pain!

In Phase 3 we'll be returning to the Forearm Plank and adding a glute isolation exercise: the Hip Abduction (see page 86).

FOREARM PLANK ON KNEES

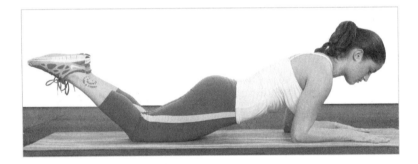

THE POSITION: Begin by lying face down on the floor. Bend your elbows and place your forearms and palms flat on the ground in front of you; your elbows should be directly underneath your shoulders and your forearms parallel to one another.

Bend your knees and lift your feet up and off the ground. Simultaneously tighten the muscles of your core and your backside (think of pulling your belly button through to your spine AND holding a $100 bill between your glute cheeks) while your push your upper body up and off the ground.

Maintain a straight line from the back of your neck to your knees and hold as long as you can. Aim to increase your time each workout.

FOREARM PLANK ON TOES

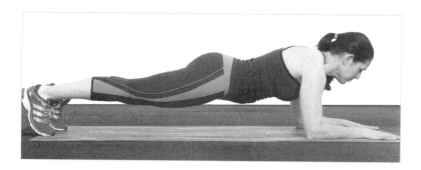

THE POSITION: Begin by lying face down on the floor. Bend your elbows and place your forearms and palms flat on the ground in front of you; your elbows should be directly underneath your shoulders and your forearms parallel to one another.

Extend your legs straight behind you, approximately hip-distance apart, with your toes on the ground. Contracting the muscles of your core and rear end, push your entire body up and off the ground, balancing yourself on your forearms and the balls of your feet.

Maintain a straight line from the back of your neck to your heels and hold as long as you can. If you find your hips sagging or your butt up in the air, you've lost your perfect form and it's time to take a break. Aim to increase your time each workout.

Step-Ups

Step-ups are a great exercise for developing single-leg quad and glute strength. They require balance, concentration, and good kinesthetic awareness. Focus on using just the bench leg to do the work, avoiding the temptation to push off with the floor leg. Resisting gravity during the eccentric part of the contraction will further increase the efficacy of the move. Be aware of any tendency your knees have to swerve inward or outward during the working phase of this exercise.

Beginners will start by using body weight only. Once you've mastered the movement, add weight to the exercise by either holding dumbbells at your sides (Intermediate) or a barbell across your shoulders (Advanced).

STEP-UP

This exercise can also be done with a weight bench or low step.

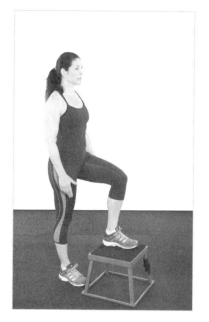

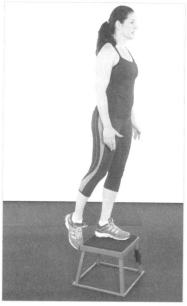

WEIGHTED VARIATION: Intermediate and Advanced exercisers can increase the challenge of this exercise by either holding a pair of dumbbells at their sides or by resting a barbell across both shoulders.

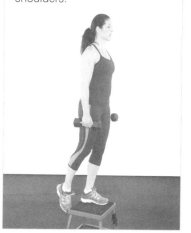

1 Stand facing a plyo box. Place your left foot on top of the plyo box and bring your right foot close to the bench. Your feet should be approximately hip-width apart.

2 Standing tall, with your shoulders back and down and eyes forward, contract your abs, glutes, and quads. Push through the left (bench foot) heel to pull yourself up to standing atop the plyo box, left leg fully extended, right leg trailing behind. Focus on keeping the left knee from pulling inward or splaying outward.

Bend the left knee and slowly lower your right leg to the floor. If you're finding it a challenge not to push off with your floor leg, keep the right foot flexed so that the sole just touches the floor between reps.

Perform all repetitions on the left side before switching legs.

Hip Extensions

One of the functions of the hamstrings is hip extension; straightening the hips when rising from a squat or pulling up on the return phase of a dead lift. Performing isolated hip extensions either on the floor or using a back extension machine can further increase the strength of not only your hamstrings, but also your glutes and lower back.

Beginners will practice this move on the floor. Intermediate and Advanced exercisers will progress to the back extension machine, perfecting the movement with body weight only before adding load to the exercise by holding a weight plate across their chest throughout the exercise. Avoid curling the upper back under at the bottom of the movement and hyperextending the lower back at the end. Maintaining a straight line from your heels to the back of your head is the safest way to start and finish the exercise.

LYING HIP EXTENSION

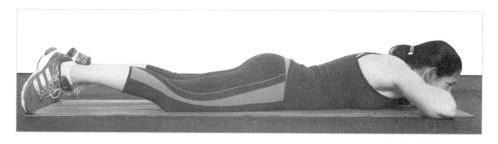

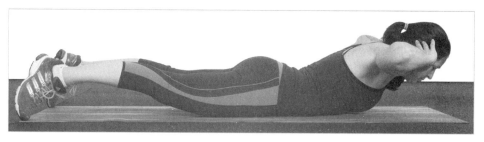

1 Begin by laying face down on a mat with your feet hip-distance apart and hands placed either on the floor beside your head or with your fingers behind your ears.

2 Contract your abdominals and glutes to raise your torso up and off the mat. Hold for 2 to 3 seconds before slowly lowering yourself back to the starting position.

To avoid placing undue stress on your lower spine, avoid hyperextending your back.

HIP EXTENSION

You should feel this exercise primarily in the lower back, glutes, and hamstrings. If you feel like your quads and calves are doing most of the work, try relaxing them; your body weight will not cause the machine to tip forward (even if your brain tells you that it might).

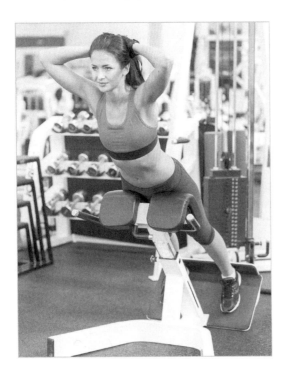

1 Position yourself in the back extension machine, with your feet hooked under the leg anchors and hips extending just above the padded hip rest. Placing your arms behind your head and contracting your abdominals to maintain a neutral arch in your spine, lower your upper body as far as you comfortably can.

2 Squeeze your glutes and lift your torso until it's in line with your legs; avoid coming up too high and placing unnecessary pressure on your lower spine.

3 Pause, then slowly lower your torso back to the starting position.

WEIGHTED VARIATION:
Perform a Hip Extension as described above, but hold a weight plate tightly against your chest.

Hip Abduction

Phase 3 includes the addition of an isolation exercise targeting the glute medius. Rather than use the Abductor/Adductor machine—many gyms don't have one, and even if yours does, you probably don't feel very comfortable using it—we'll perform them first from a side lying position, using dumbbells to weight the move (Beginners), and then from a standing position, either using resistance tubing or a cable and pulley machine (Intermediate and Advanced).

Phase 3 also progresses the Forearm Plank on Toes (page 77) by adding a hip abduction movement. Beginners will perform this exercise without weights, focusing on slow, controlled movements and maintaining proper plank form. Intermediate and Advanced lifters can add load to the exercise by attaching either an anchored resistance band or the cushioned strap of a cable and pulley machine around their ankles. Both levels of the exercise require that you be able to plank on your toes. If you've been consistent with this program, even those who had to plank from the knees during Phase 1, should be strong enough to hold a toe plank for the 6 to 8 reps required.

WEIGHTED LYING LEG RAISE

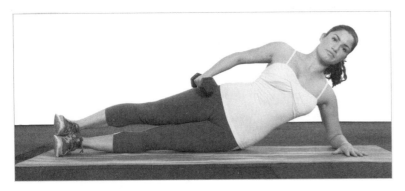

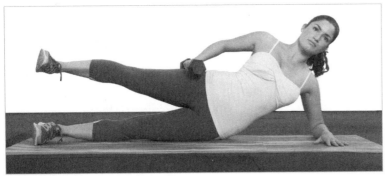

1 Lay on a mat, on your side. Your legs should be extended straight out, with shoulders, hips, and ankles all in a line. You can either rest your head on the mat or raise yourself up on your forearm and support your head with your hand. Holding a dumbbell against the side of your top leg, flex the foot.

2 Without moving any other part of your body, lift your leg as high as you can.

Pause, then return the leg to starting position, without letting your feet touch between repetitions; doing so gives the gluteus medius a rest too frequently for the exercise to be effective.

Complete all repetitions on one side before switching to the other.

STANDING CABLE HIP ABDUCTION

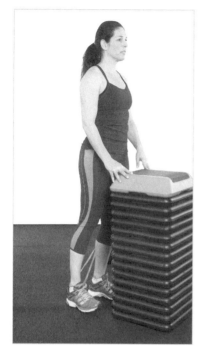

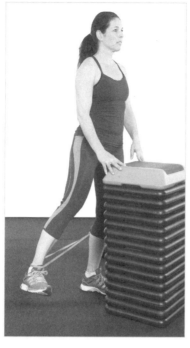

1 Loop an anchored resistance band around your right ankle.

Standing with your left side facing the anchor point and holding on to a vertical support (or pillar of step risers, as pictured here) with both hands, flex your right foot and lift it up and off the floor.

2 Keeping both legs nearly straight and without moving your upper body, lift your right leg out and to the side as far as you can.

Slowly return to the starting position, keeping your muscles under tension for the entire set.

Complete all repetitions on the right side before switching sides.

CABLE-AND-PULLEY MACHINE VARIATION: Attach an ankle strap to the low pulley of a cable and pulley machine. Wrap the strap around your right ankle. Standing with your left side facing the weight stack and holding on to the vertical support with your left hand, cross your right leg in front of your left. Keeping both legs nearly straight and without moving your upper body, lift your right leg out and to the side as far as you can.

Slowly return to the starting position. Don't let the weights rest on the weight stack between repetitions; keep your muscles under tension for the entire set.

Complete all repetitions on the right before switching sides.

FOREARM PLANK WITH HIP ABDUCTION

Don't rush through this exercise; the longer it takes you to complete the hip abductions, the longer you'll be holding your plank. Time under tension is what we need to build muscle and get stronger; don't cheat yourself by hurrying.

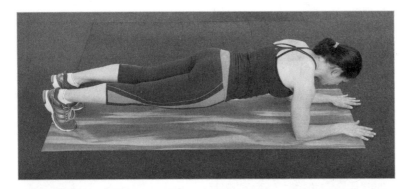

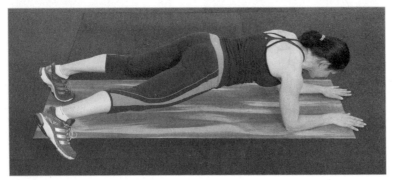

1 Assume a Forearm Plank on Toes (page 77), with weight evenly distributed on your forearms and toes.

2 Keeping your hips low and pointed toward the ground, flex your right foot and lift your toes about 2 inches off the ground.

Squeeze your glutes and move your right leg out to the side of your body; the leg should stay the same distance from the floor throughout the movement, with the toes pointing downward the entire time.

Return the leg to starting position and repeat until all repetitions are complete.

Switch legs and start again.

FOREARM PLANK WITH WEIGHTED HIP ABDUCTION

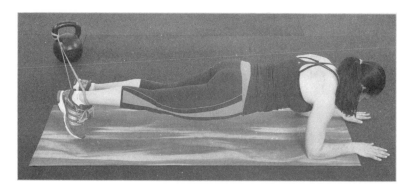

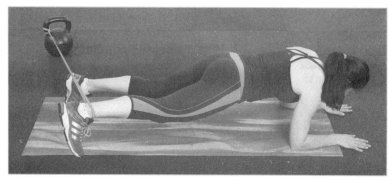

1 If using a resistance band, loop one end of the band around a post or through the handle of a heavy kettlebell (as pictured) and anchor it by slipping one handle through the other. Secure the free handle around your right foot. If using a cable and pulley machine, attach the cushioned strap to the lowest vertical position. Wrap it around your right ankle and tighten to ensure a snug fit.

Assume a Forearm Plank on Toes (page 77) with the resistance band anchor or cable-and-pulley machine on the left side of your body. Make sure that you're far enough from the pole to have already created some tension on the band and are far enough from the machine to have lifted the weight up slightly off the stack.

2 Lift your right leg 5 to 6 inches off the ground and flex your foot to keep your toes pointing downward. Squeeze your glutes and move the leg outward and away from the body.

Slowly return to starting position before beginning the next repetition.

Complete all reps on the right side, then repeat on the other side.

Tabata Options

In order to maximize the benefits of a Tabata workout, the exercise used needs to be able to elevate your heart rate within just a few repetitions. Done properly and at near maximal intensity, each of the following three options should leave you begging for a rest by the time you've finished a mere 20 seconds of work. If not, push a little bit harder on the next interval.

BURPEES

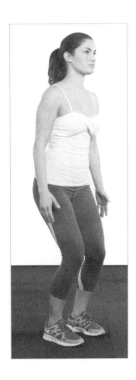 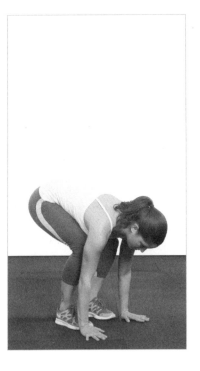 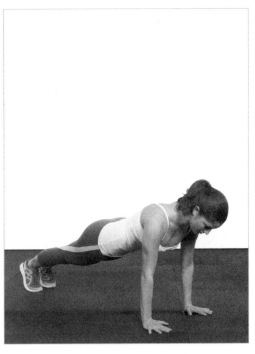

1 Start by standing with your feet hip-distance apart, hands at your sides.

2 Place your hands on the ground directly in front of your feet.

3 Jump feet back, landing in a high plank position.

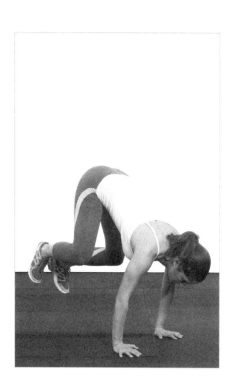
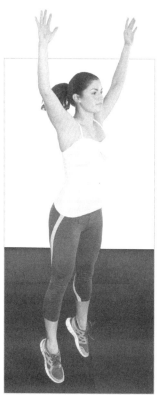

4–5 Immediately jump your feet back up to your hands and explode upward, reaching your hands toward the ceiling. Repeat with as little rest between repetitions as possible. Beginners may make this move easier by choosing to step their feet back into the plank. Advanced exercisers can challenge themselves further by dropping their chest all the way to the floor, rather than remaining in high plank.

SQUAT JUMPS

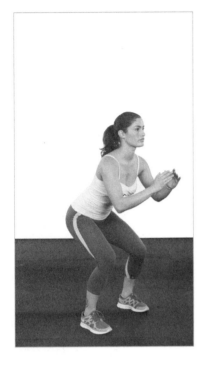 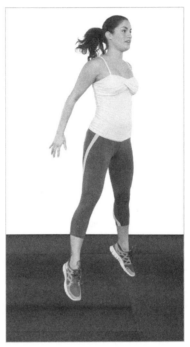

1 Standing with your feet slightly wider than your hips, toes facing forward, drop down into a Bodyweight Squat.

2 Explode upward by pushing through the heels, "catching air" at the top of the movement.

Land softly, with knees slightly bent, and immediately begin the next repetition. Hands can be held at your sides, swung forward and back to help with the jumps, or placed behind your head ("prisoner" style) to further engage the core.

SPLIT SQUAT JUMPS

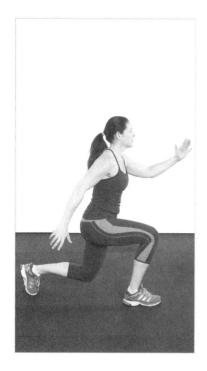 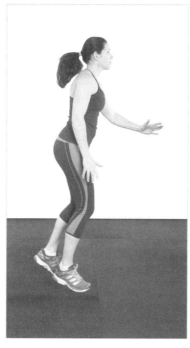 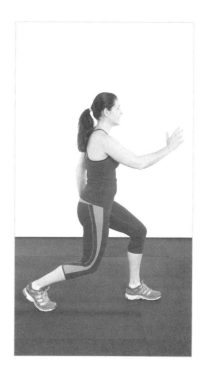

1 Assume a split (or lunge) stance, one leg behind the other, with your feet approximately hip-distance apart. Lower your back knee toward the floor, into a lunge, keeping front knee behind the toes and torso erect.

2 Explode upward, switching front and back legs in mid-air.

3 Land softly and continue alternating legs for the duration of the interval. Hands can be held at your sides, swung forward and back to help with the jumps, or placed behind your head to further engage the core.

SPEED SKATERS

To make this exercise more challenging, try jumping farther, swinging your arms more forcefully, and remaining as low to the ground as you can.

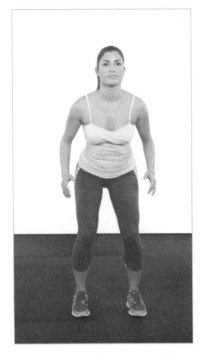 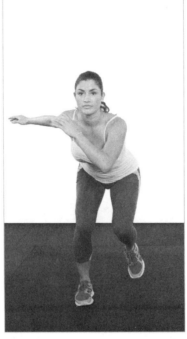 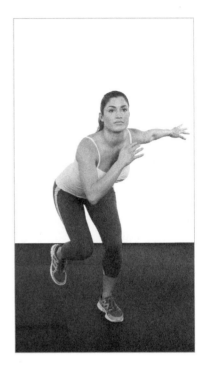

1 Stand with your feet hip-width apart, arms by your sides, knees bent, and upper body hinged slightly forward from the hip.

2 Engage your core and glutes before forcefully pushing off with the left leg and landing on the right.

Simultaneously sweep your left foot diagonally behind the right, and swing your left arm across the front of the body and right arm behind.

3 Reverse arm and leg movements to jump back to the left.

Continue alternating sides for the duration of the interval, attempting to minimize the amount of time your feet spend on the ground.

TWO-FOOT LATERAL HOPS

To make this exercise more challenging, try jumping over a low, stationary object like a telephone book or a step aerobics bench.

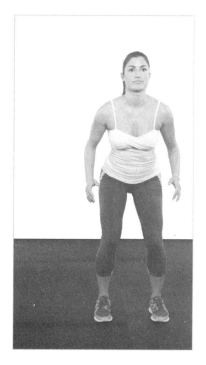 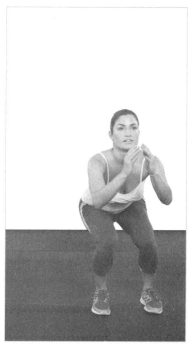 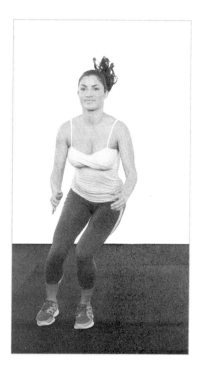

1 Start by standing with your feet together, knees slightly bent, and hands either at your sides (Beginner) or behind your head (Intermediate and Advanced).

2 Bend your knees and hinge forward slightly from the hip before springing up and to the side, landing in the same position you started from. Imagine that there's a low object that you're trying to clear, aiming to get your feet 3 to 4 inches above the ground with each hop. Always minimize impact by landing with your knees bent and abs engaged.

3 Continue alternating sides for the duration of the interval.

SIDE SHUFFLES

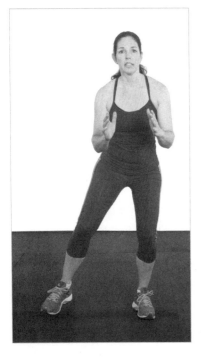 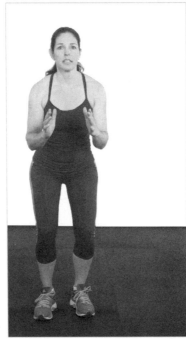 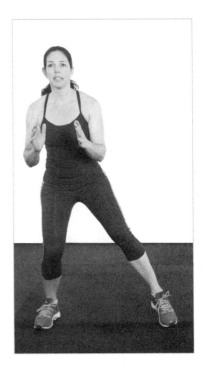

1 Start by standing with your feet together, knees slightly bent. Step your right leg out to the right.

2 Quickly bring left leg to meet the right and repeat across the length of the room and back. If you're limited for space, try shuffling 3 or 4 times to the right, then 3 or 4 times to the left. Remember to keep your abs tight and neck neutral, with eyes focused on the floor 3 or 4 feet in front of you.

3 Your arms should be held long and slightly away from the body. More advanced exercisers may choose to reach down to tap the floor with their "leading" hand before reversing the direction of the movement.

Continue for the duration of the interval.

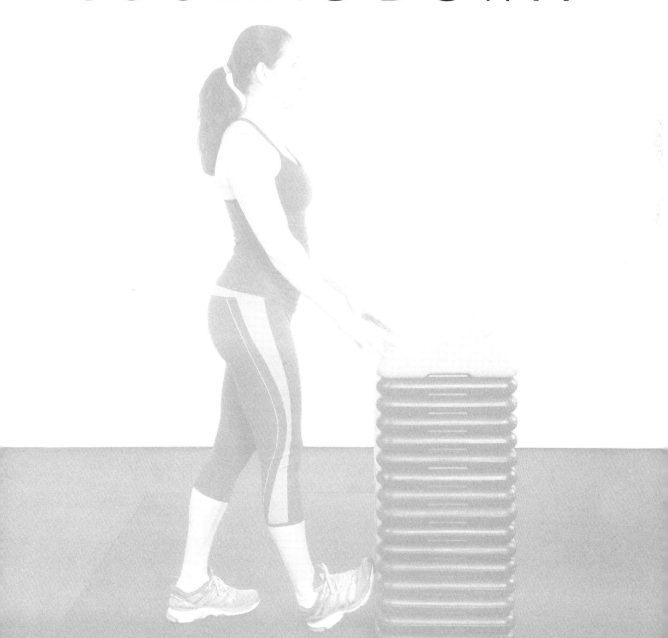

PART 4
WARMING UP AND COOLING DOWN

The Warm-Up

Before beginning any type of strenuous exercise (including the programs in this book), you need to perform a proper warm-up. Not only will it improve your workout performance, it will also help to minimize your risk of exercise-induced injury.

An effective, well-planned warm-up will physically and mentally prepare your body for exercise. It should consist of 5 to 10 minutes of continuous, mild to moderate movement and incorporate actions specific to the type of exercise to be performed. Note that the intensity of your warm-up should be significantly lower than that of your workout. Aim for an RPE of 2 or 3. Goals of the warm-up include:

Increased respiration. The function of the lungs is to provide oxygen to the muscles, tissues, and organs of your body. When we exercise, our muscles increase their demand for oxygen, a demand that must be met by increased respiration. Gradually increasing your respiration rate will allow you to continue meeting the oxygen demand of your muscles, without incurring oxygen debt and its by-product, lactic acid accumulation.

Increased blood flow. Oxygen is carried throughout the body by the blood. As respiration and oxygen uptake at the lungs increase, blood flow increases to transport oxygen to your working muscles, as well as to the heart.

Elevated heart rate. The heart serves to pump freshly oxygenated blood from the lungs to the rest of the body, as well as to pump de-oxygenated blood back to the lungs for re-oxygenation. An elevated heart rate is often the most obvious sign that your body is starting to work a bit harder as the warm-up progresses. Pay attention to how quickly your heart rate is rising and modify the intensity of your warm-up accordingly.

Increased muscle temperature. As your muscles begin to work, they increase in temperature, which decreases the work of contraction and reduces the likelihood of muscular injury.

Joint lubrication. As you begin to move your body, your brain signals the release of synovial fluid within your joints. Synovial fluid acts as a lubricant, allowing the joints to move more smoothly and through an increasingly larger range of motion as the workout proceeds.

Often, the rapid release of synovial fluid results in "cracks" and "pops" at the shoulders, knees, and ankles. As long as there is no pain involved, such sounds are of little concern.

Rehearsal of workout-specific joint movements. Performing "no load" versions of the movements in your upcoming workout acts as a rehearsal for the exercises to come. These warm-up movements gently stretch the muscles around the joints and help to generate the mind-to-muscle connection required for heavier lifting.

Improved proprioception and kinesthetic awareness. Proprioception is the awareness of the position of one's body in space. Strength training requires good proprioception and kinesthetic awareness to maximize the benefits of each exercise and to reduce the likelihood of injury. Using the warm-up to practice exercises to be performed during the actual workout enhances the mind-body connection.

While many gym-goers regularly head to the treadmill to warm up their muscles before a strength-training session, unless their workout involves more time on the treadmill, they haven't properly prepared their body for the work to come.

Why? Warm-ups need to be specific to the exercises about to be performed. The programs in *Ultimate Booty Workouts* include squats, lunges, dead lifts, lateral lunges, and hip thrusts. Hence, we need to warm up the muscles responsible for those movements and the joints at which those movements occur.

The following body-weight warm-up routine will take your hips, knees, and ankles through all of their normal planes of motion while simultaneously raising your body temperature, elevating your heart rate, and preparing you mentally for the workout to come. In addition, several of the moves will serve to "turn on" your glutes and core muscles, both of which will increase the efficacy of the workouts themselves.

Expect to spend 5 to 10 minutes moving through the 12 exercises in the order described, concentrating on increasing your range of motion with each repetition. All movements should be fluid and controlled: no bouncing! Detailed instructions for each exercise are provided below.

Body-Weight Warm-Up Routine

EXERCISE	REPS	TEMPO
1. Narrow Marches p. 98	20	moderate
2. Wide Marches p. 98	20	moderate
3. Walk-Out Planks p. 99	10	moderate
4. Alternating Knee Hugs p. 99	10 each side	slow
5. Narrow Squats p. 100	10	slow
6. Wide Squats p. 100	10	slow
7. Plié Squats p. 101	10	slow
8. Jumping Jacks p.101	20	fast
9. Alternating Forward Lunges p. 102	10 each side	slow
10. Alternating Curtsey Lunges p. 102	10 each side	slow
11. Alternating Hamstring Curls p. 103	10 each side	moderate
12. Alternating-Leg Lateral Band Walk p. 103	10 each side	moderate

NARROW MARCHES

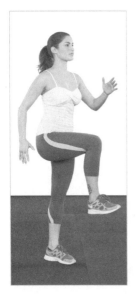 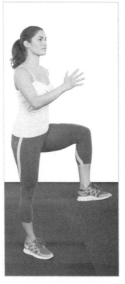

THE MOVEMENT: Stand with your feet under your hips and arms at your sides. March in place by alternately lifting one knee up to waist height and swinging your arms front to back. Concentrate on increasing your range of motion and breathing with the movement.

WIDE MARCHES

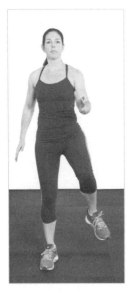 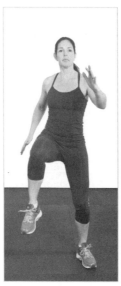

THE MOVEMENT: Stand with your feet wider than hip-width apart and toes pointing forward. March in place by alternately lifting one knee up to waist height and swinging your arms front to back, bending your elbows and pumping your arms to help raise the knees. Concentrate on increasing your range of motion and breathing with the movement.

WALK-OUT PLANKS

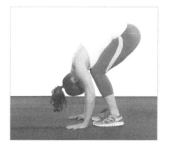 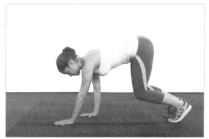 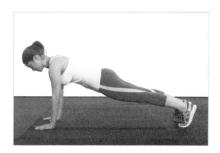

1 Stand tall with your feet under your hips and arms at your sides. Reach your hands down toward your feet, bending your knees slightly if necessary.

2–3 Walk your hands out in front of you, lowering your body into a high plank position, ending with your hands directly under your shoulders and back straight. Walk your hands back in toward your feet and return to standing, exaggerating a tall posture with your shoulders back and down at the end of the movement.

ALTERNATING KNEE HUGS

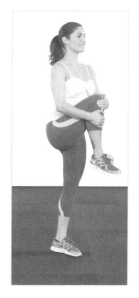 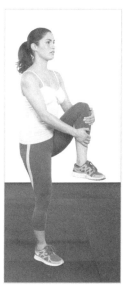

1 Stand tall with your feet hip-width apart and arms at your sides. Balancing on one foot, lift the opposite knee up toward your chest, wrapping your arms around your shin to hug the knee in close to your body.

2 Pause before slowly lowering the foot to the ground and repeating on the other side.

Continue alternating sides until all repetitions are complete.

NARROW SQUATS

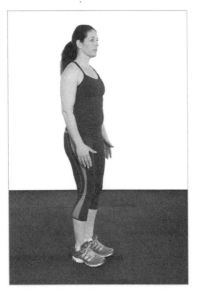 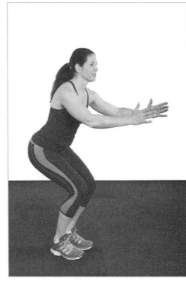

1 Stand with your feet hip-width apart and arms at your sides.

2 Sit back into a shallow squat, with your butt reaching behind you and knees remaining behind your toes. Reach your arms out in front of you to counterbalance the backward movement of the hips.

Return to standing by pushing through your heels and pulling your hands back in toward your body.

Complete all repetitions slowly and with increasing depth as the quads and glutes "wake up."

WIDE SQUATS

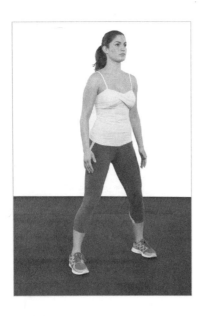 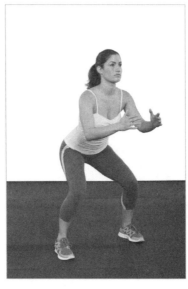

1 Stand with your feet placed slightly wider than hip-width apart and toes pointing forward or slightly turned out.

2 Sit back into a shallow squat, with your butt reaching behind you and knees remaining behind your toes. Reach your arms out in front of you to counterbalance the backward movement of the hips.

Return to standing by pushing through your heels and pulling your hands back in toward your body.

Complete all repetitions slowly and with increasing depth as the quads and glutes "wake up."

PLIÉ SQUATS

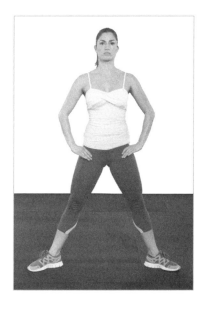
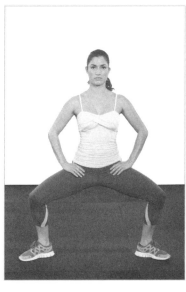

1 Stand with your feet wide apart and toes turned out to 10 and 2 o'clock.

2 Drop your butt down toward the floor by bending your knees and ankles, but without hinging forward from the hip.

Push through your heels, squeeze your glutes, and draw your inner thighs toward one another to return to standing.

Gradually increase the depth of the squat as you progress through the warm-up.

JUMPING JACKS

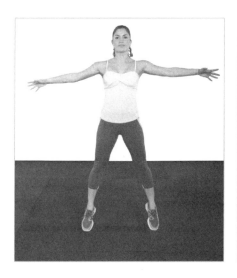
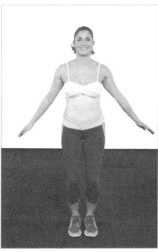

1 Stand with your feet together and hands by your sides. Simultaneously jump your legs out wide and raise your arms to shoulder height.

2 Jump legs back together and lower arms to the starting position.

Continue until all repetitions are complete, slowly increasing range of motion and speed as appropriate.

ALTERNATING FORWARD LUNGES

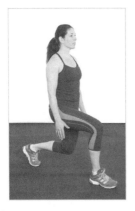 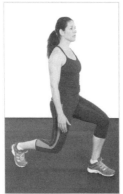

1 Stand with your feet shoulder-width apart and arms at your sides. Step forward with your right leg and lower yourself into a lunge. Your back knee should drop straight down and form a 90-degree angle with the floor.

2 Push through the right heel to return to the starting position. Repeat on the left side and continue alternating sides until all repetitions are complete.

To avoid knee pain, ensure that your front knee is not extending beyond your toes. If so, try taking a slightly larger step forward.

ALTERNATING CURTSEY LUNGES

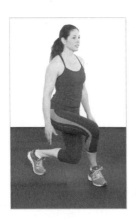 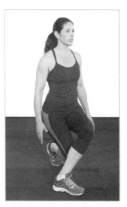

1 Stand with your feet shoulder-width apart and hands at your sides or on your hips. Cross your right foot in front of your left, stepping about a foot to the left of your left foot. Bend both knees and lower your back knee toward the floor, as if you're curtseying to the queen.

2 Push through your front foot to return to the starting position. Repeat the movement on the other side, alternating right and left sides until all repetitions are complete. Make sure that hips and shoulders remain facing forward throughout, with your torso tall and abdominals engaged.

ALTERNATING HAMSTRING CURLS

Be sure to fully extend your arms between reps to maximize the benefit of the movement.

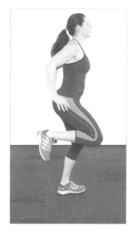 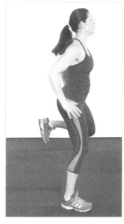

1 Stand with your feet slightly wider than shoulder-width apart. Bend your knees slightly and lean your torso forward, extending your arms out in front of you at shoulder height. Simultaneously pull your arms back toward your body and curl your right heel up toward your buttocks.

2 Extend your arms, lower your foot, and repeat on the left side.

Continue alternating sides until all repetitions are complete, focusing on keeping your abs and glutes tight and eyes focused forward.

ALTERNATING-LEG LATERAL BAND WALK

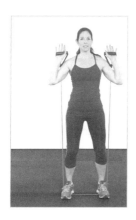 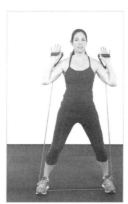

1 Start by standing on a resistance band with your knees slightly bent and feet shoulder-width apart. Bringing the band up and behind your arms, hold the handles at shoulder height to create tension on the band.

2 Keeping your knees slightly bent, step sideways with your right leg, thereby increasing the tension on the band, before stepping your left foot in toward the right and returning to starting position.

Reverse the movement; step sideways with your left leg and bring your right foot in toward the left.

Continue alternating which leg leads until all repetitions are complete, making sure to keep tension on the band for the duration of the set.

The Cool-Down

At the end of an intense workout, it's necessary to slowly return the body to its pre-workout state to avoid feelings of dizziness and fatigue. When we stop a vigorous exercise session abruptly, blood pools in the lower limbs. With reduced circulation, cardiac output decreases and lightheadedness may occur. Because muscle movement helps to pump blood back to the heart, it's important to continue with lower intensity physical activity after the last strength training set or Tabata interval is complete.

In addition to preventing you from "seeing stars," adding 5 or 6 minutes of light cardiovascular movement to the end of your strength training program may also help dissipate any lactic acid buildup and reduce the intensity of delayed onset muscle soreness (DOMS). Try hopping on an exercise bike, elliptical trainer, or rowing machine, walking on the treadmill, or taking a nice, easy stroll around the block. By the time you've finished, your heart rate will have returned to normal and your muscles will be ready for the final two components of your workout: foam rolling and stretching.

Foam Rolling

In a perfect world, we'd all have access to post-workout massage. Strong hands to eliminate the knots and kinks in our muscles that weight training sometimes triggers. While a post-workout massage might not be in your budget, a foam roller—the next best thing—most certainly is!

Typically made of hard plastic and covered with foam, cylindrical foam rollers come in a variety of lengths and densities. The denser the foam, the more pressure applied to the muscle and the less "comfortable" the experience. I always recommend that my clients start with a fairly soft roller and work their way up to the more dense variety as they become more familiar with its use (and accustomed to the associated discomfort).

Massaging your limbs with a foam roller not only loosens tight muscles, it also breaks up any scar tissue (or muscular "adhesions") that might be preventing the muscle from performing optimally. Improvements in range of motion and reductions in DOMS have also been documented. Chronic muscle tightness is a recipe for injury; think of foam rolling as preventative maintenance, and make it a regular part of your workout.

After completing your *Ultimate Booty Workouts*, you'll need to roll your hamstrings and glutes. If you're feeling tightness in your quadriceps or calves, foam roll them as well. Plan on spending a minute or 2 per muscle group per leg. See below for tips and tricks for rolling each body part.

GLUTEUS MAXIMUS

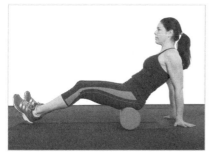

1 Position your foam roller so that its long axis is perpendicular to your body. Take a seat on top, with your legs extended in front of you and hands on the floor behind your back.

2 Using your hands and feet to both support and guide you, move your body forward and backward over the roller, making sure to cover the entire muscle from the top of your hamstrings to the bottom of your lower back.

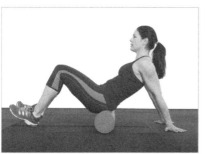

Aim for slow, steady movement and spend extra time anywhere you feel intense discomfort (a sure sign of extreme muscle tightness).

To increase the pressure and work one side of the body at a time, bend both legs at the knees and place one ankle across the opposite knee. Use the arms and single supporting leg to roll your gluteal muscle.

GLUTEUS MEDIUS

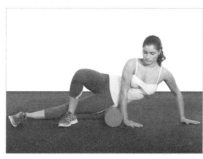

1 Position your foam roller so that its long axis is perpendicular to your body. Take a seat on top, with your legs extended in front of you and hands on the floor behind your back. Turn your body slightly to the left so that your left hip and outside of the upper thigh are now in contact with the roller. Cross your right leg over your left so that your right foot is flat on the floor. Take your right hand and place it on the floor in front of your left.

2 Using your hands and right foot for support and guidance, slowly move your body up and down the roller, covering the area from waist to mid-thigh.

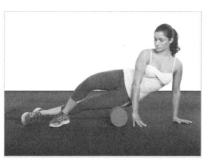

If you feel tightness in the outer thigh area, you may want to continue rolling all the way down to the outside of the knee. Many people have tight iliotibial (IT) bands, which can lead to knee injuries if left unchecked.

Repeat on the right side.

HAMSTRINGS

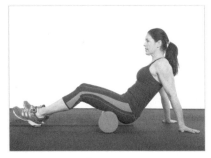

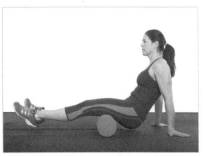

1 Position your foam roller so that its long axis is perpendicular to your body. Take a seat on top, with your legs extended in front of you and hands on the floor behind your back.

2 Using your hands for guidance and support, move your body back slightly, so that the roller is just behind the upper hamstring. Continue moving your body backward to apply pressure to the hamstring from just below the glutes all the way down to the back of the knee. Return to the top and repeat.

Because the hamstring is a long muscle, it can be awkward to roll its entire length in one smooth movement. It's just as effective to roll in sections: roll the top half of the muscle several times, then reposition your body and repeat along the bottom half.

QUADRICEPS

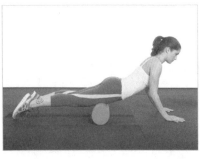

1 Turn face down and position the roller underneath the tops of your thighs. Point your toes and press your feet together, and lift your feet up and off the ground. Place your forearms on the floor with your elbows directly under your shoulders, and shift your weight slightly forward.

2 Using your forearms to guide and support you, move your body forward and backward, rolling from the top of the left thigh to just above the knee cap.

CALVES

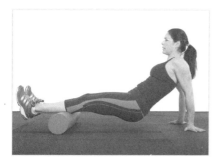

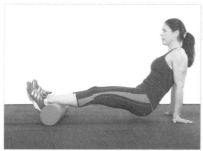

1 Position your foam roller so that its long axis is perpendicular to your body. Take a seat on top, with your legs extended in front of you and hands on the floor behind your back. Move your body until the roller is directly under your calves.

2 Begin by rolling both calves at once, from just above the ankle to just below the knee.

If you require additional pressure, cross one ankle over the other and focus on rolling one leg at a time.

Stretching

In addition to strength and cardiovascular training, flexibility training is one of the key components of a balanced exercise program. Flexibility, defined as the range of motion in a joint, is best improved by stretching.

A well-designed workout will incorporate both dynamic and static stretching, stretching with and without movement, respectively. Studies show that dynamic stretching is best performed as part of the pre-exercise warm-up. Most of the range-of-motion warm-up exercises described in this book are in fact, dynamic stretches.

Static stretching appears to be best for long-term increases in joint range of motion and is most effective when performed at the end of your workout, when muscles are warm and blood supply to the muscles is plentiful. Not only does post-exercise stretching improve the range of motion in our joints, it may also contribute to:

Decreased muscular tension and soreness post-exercise. Stretching promotes muscular relaxation. When our muscles are in a constant state of tension or contraction, more energy is required for movement and activity. Chronic muscular tension can result in pain and injury.

Better posture. Tight hip flexors and hamstrings can pull your pelvis forward, contributing to postural deviations, including kyphosis. Gentle post-workout stretching can help to lengthen shortened muscles and contribute to better overall muscular balance.

Improved circulation. Regular stretching can enhance the circulation of blood and nutrients to the joints, thereby allowing greater elasticity of tissues and more freedom of movement.

Reduced risk of injury. Although there is insufficient data to support this conclusion, many fitness professionals believe that increasing a joint's ROM via stretching will result in decreased tissue resistance, thereby reducing the likelihood of any particular exercise exceeding a joint's natural range of motion and becoming injured.

Relaxation and increased enjoyment. For many people, the time they spend on their mat post-exercise is the most enjoyable part of a workout. Holding stretches and focusing on breath-ing through the stretch relaxes both the body and the mind and often generates an overall feeling of well-being and contentment.

To ensure that you're getting the most out of your post-workout stretch, follow the guidelines below:

Perform all stretches slowly, with control, and below the threshold of pain. Pain is your body's way of protecting you from injury. Honor it and reduce the intensity of the stretch just a bit.

Hold each stretch long enough to allow the muscle to relax. Aim for 15 to 30 seconds, although the longer a stretch is held, the more relaxed the muscle becomes and the greater the potential for long-term lengthening. Don't ever worry that you're stretching too much; I've never met anyone guilty of that!

Focus on the muscle you're trying to stretch and concentrate on relaxing it. Stretching may be a static exercise, but it still requires physical and mental engagement to reap the most benefits.

Avoid bouncing or "ballistic" stretches. These kinds of stretches can place undue strain on the joint and damage muscles, tendons, and ligaments.

Don't hold your breath. Exhale into the stretch and breathe slowly and rhythmically while holding it. Concentrate on feeling your rib cage expand and contract.

If a muscle is particularly tight, stretch it in stages. Find your "edge" (the point at which your body resists) and hold for 15 to 30 seconds. Take a deep breath in, and as you exhale, take the stretch a bit deeper, finding the next "edge" before holding again.

Make sure to stretch both sides of the body, for example the left and right hamstrings.

Post-Exercise Stretching Routine Suggestions

As with the warm-up exercises, it's important that your post-exercise stretches target the specific muscles worked during your strength training sessions.

Below you'll find some suggestions for stretching your hamstrings, gluteals, lower back, calves, and quadriceps. Make sure you choose at least one stretch for each muscle group. Performing an extra stretch or two for any muscle group that's particularly tight is highly recommended.

Note that many of these stretches target multiple muscles; for example, the Seated Hamstring Stretch will also stretch the gluteals on the opposite side while the Seated Spinal Twist will stretch the gluteals, erector spinae, and obliques. Focus on stretching the target muscle, but notice where else on your body you feel the stretch.

LYING HAMSTRING

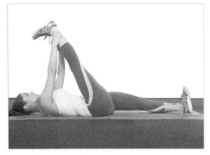

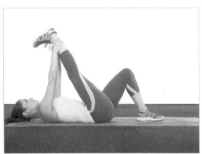

1 Lie on your back, with your legs extended long on the floor and arms at your sides. Lift your right leg up until your ankle is directly above your hip. Flex your foot to straighten your leg (without locking the knee), reach your hands around your calf and gently pull the leg in toward your chest.

2 If you feel your lower back lifting off the ground, bend your left leg and place your left foot flat on the floor.

Repeat on the other side.

SEATED HAMSTRING

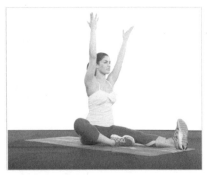

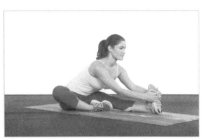

1 Sit on your mat with both legs extended straight out in front of you and hands extended upward. Bend your right knee and place your right foot against the inside of your left thigh, just above the knee joint.

2 With your torso tall, hinge at your hips to lower your chest down toward your left thigh by either holding on to your foot or placing your hands on the floor on either side of your leg to support your upper body during the stretch. Make sure that you're not rounding through the back by keeping shoulders retracted and chest aimed forward.

Repeat on the other side.

STANDING HAMSTRING

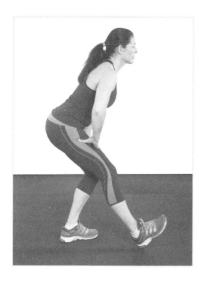

THE POSITION: From a standing position, extend your straightened right leg out about 12 inches in front of you. Flex your right ankle to pull your toes up and off the floor. Keeping your torso tall and your back flat, hinge forward from the hip until you feel a stretch up the backside of your right leg. Place your hands on your right thigh to support your upper body and hold the stretch.

Repeat with the other leg.

LYING KNEE HUG

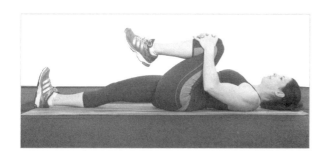

THE POSITION: Start by lying on your back, legs extended straight out on the floor and arms by your sides. Bend your left leg and wrap your arms around your shin to pull your left thigh in toward your chest. Concentrate on keeping your right leg straight and in contact with the ground.

Switch sides and repeat.

LYING FIGURE FOUR

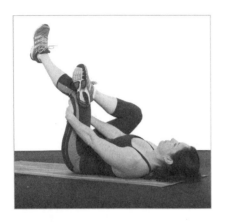

THE POSITION: Begin by lying on your back with both knees bent and feet flat on the floor. Place your right foot on your left thigh, just above the knee. Reach your hands around your left thigh, clasping them together behind it to draw both legs in toward your chest. Concentrate on keeping the right hip open by pulling back slightly on the right knee.

Unwind and repeat on the other side.

SEATED SPINAL TWIST

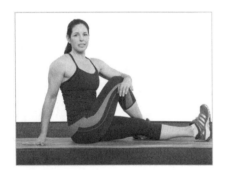

THE POSITION: From a seated position, extend your left leg out straight in front of you. Cross your right leg over the left, placing your right foot on the floor on the outside of your left thigh. Place the palm of your left hand on the outside of your right knee. Your right hand will be on the floor beside you or slightly behind your midline. Lift through the torso to create length before turning your upper body to the right and looking over your right shoulder. Use your left hand to increase the intensity of the twist.

Move slowly out of the twist and repeat on the other side.

CAT LIFT–COW TUCK

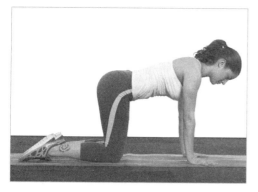

1 Come onto all fours with your hands directly under your shoulders and knees under your hips. Your back will be straight; your toes may be tucked or untucked, as you wish.

2 As you breathe in, drop you head down between your arms and round your back up toward the ceiling. Concentrate on feeling the expansion in your rib cage and the stretch in your lower and mid-back.

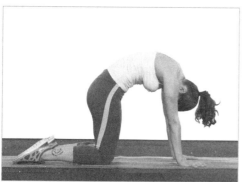

3 Exhale as you return to the starting position and move through it by raising your head and looking forward while you simultaneously create a convex curve through your lower back.

Continue moving your body through the lift and tuck, matching the movements to your breathing.

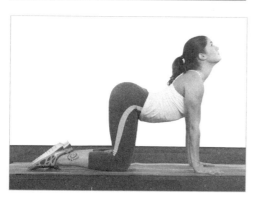

CHILD'S POSE

This classic yoga pose adds hand variations to maximize the lower back stretch.

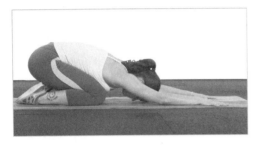

1 Starting on all fours, with your knees under your hips and toes untucked, sit back so that your butt is resting on your heels. Extend your arms straight out in front of you and lower your forehead to the floor.

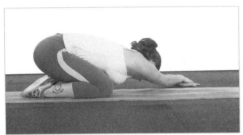

2 After you've held this position for 30 seconds, walk both hands over to the top left corner of your mat, making sure not to lose the contact between heels and glutes. Feel the stretch all down the right side of your body, including your right hip and outer thigh.

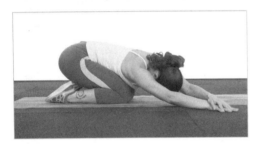

3 Walk hands to the top right corner of your mat and hold again.

STRAIGHT-LEG CALF

This calf stretch focuses on the gastrocnemius, which assists the hamstrings in knee flexion.

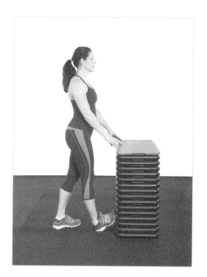

THE POSITION: Stand facing a wall or countertop. Placing the ball of your right foot against the wall, straighten your right leg and lean forward slightly until you feel a stretch in the back of your leg. Place your hands on the wall or countertop for support. Hold for 15 to 30 seconds before switching sides.

BENT-LEG CALF

This calf stretch focuses on the soleus, which assists the hamstrings in knee flexion.

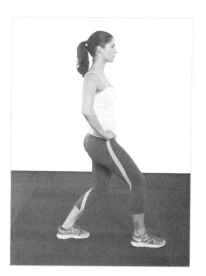

THE POSITION: Start by standing with your feet hip-width apart, hands on your thighs or hips. Take a small step back with your left foot. Keeping your toes pointed forward and both heels on the ground, bend your knees as you lower your left knee down toward the floor. Concentrate on keeping your torso upright and your right hip pressed forward. Stop when you feel the stretch in the back of your lower leg. Step your feet back together and repeat on the right side.

STANDING HIP FLEXOR

This quad stretch requires that you be comfortable balancing on one leg. If you're "balance challenged," make sure there's a wall or stable chair nearby to place your free hand on while you stretch.

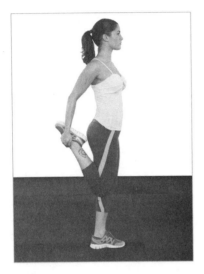

THE POSITION: While standing on your left leg, reach your right hand around and behind you to grab your right foot by either the ankle or the shoelaces. Pull the right foot up toward your butt, keeping your knees as close together as you can and pushing forward with your right hip flexor. Maintain a slight bend in the left leg and hold for 15 to 30 seconds.

Repeat the stretch on the other leg.

SIDE-LYING SINGLE-LEG HIP FLEXOR

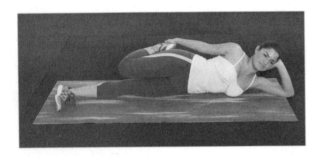

THE POSITION: Lie on left your side, hips stacked one on top of the other, legs long, and upper body supported on the forearm closest to the floor. Engage through your core, bend your right leg at the knee, and reach your right hand behind you to grab your right foot either at the ankle or by the shoelaces. Like you did for the Standing Hip Flexor, concentrate on keeping your knees close together and pushing forward with the right hip flexor. Hold for 15 to 30 seconds, then release.

Roll over and repeat the stretch on the other side.

APPENDIX

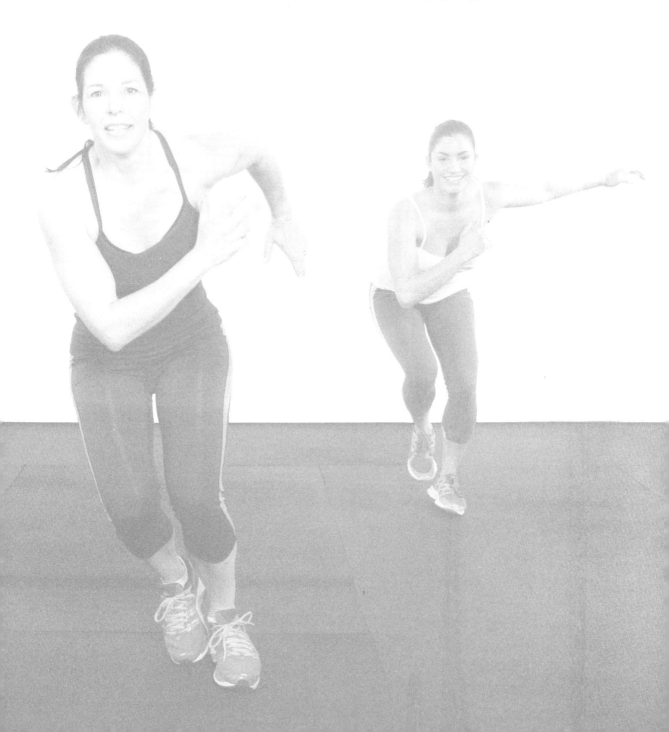

Blank Workout Templates

Use the charts in this section to track your workout progress. Make one photocopy for each workout. Record the exercise name, the weight you used, the number of reps you performed for each set, and how you felt during and after your workout. See the filled-in example below.

Phase 1: Setting the Foundation

Date: _1-15-2014_

EXERCISE	REPS	WEIGHT	COMMENTS
1. Ball squat	15/13/12 (in sets 1, 2, and 3)	10 pounds	Heavier weights next time
2. Stationary lunge	15/13/12 (R & L sides)	No weights	Dumbbells next time
3. Hamstring curl on ball	12/11/8	n/a	These are hard!
4. Plié squat	15/15/15	10 pounds	Heavier weights next time
5. Lateral band walk	15/15/15	n/a	Progress to lateral lunges
6. Glute bridge	12/12/11	No weights	These burned!
7. Plank on forearms & knees	30 sec/ 25 sec/ 35 sec	No weights	Aim for 40 sec next time

Phase 1: Setting the Foundation   Date: _____

EXERCISE	REPS	WEIGHT	COMMENTS
1.			
2.			
3.			
4.			
5.			
6.			
7.			

Phase 2: Building Muscle (Hypertrophy)

Date: _____

Workout #_____

EXERCISE	REPS	WEIGHT	COMMENTS
1a.			
1b.			
2a.			
2b.			
3a.			
3b.			
Optional HIIT (exercise, cycle lengths, total time)			

Phase 3: Leaning and Cutting

Date: _____

Workout #_____

EXERCISE	REPS	WEIGHT	COMMENTS
1			
2a.			
2b.			
3a.			
3b.			
Tabata (exercise, cycles, total time)			

Index

Acknowledgments

When I finished writing the manuscript for the *Ultimate Booty Workouts*, I thought that the hardest part of the project was behind me. Not so. Turns out that the most difficult part of writing a book is thanking everyone who was involved in its creation. Thanking them honestly and authentically and making sure that you haven't left anybody out!

Because my memory works linearly, I've chosen to express my gratitude to friends, family, and colleagues chronologically. Just because your name is near the bottom of the list doesn't mean you haven't had an enormous impact on the outcome of this project.

Thank you acquisitions editor Kelly Reed and managing editor Claire Chun at Ulysses Press for trusting me with this project. I'm so grateful for the opportunity to write for your readers and to share my love of strength training with women all over North America.

Thanks to Carla Birnberg, writer, community-builder, self-esteem ninja, and honorary sister, for sending Kelly my way when she first approached you about writing this book. Your willingness to share opportunities, ideas, vulnerabilities, and the minutia of everyday life is truly treasured.

Thank you Bernie Crespi, husband, child-wrangler, idea-bouncer-offer, and deliverer of morning coffee, for your constant love and support and for not sharing your daily word count with me on days when I found writing difficult.

Thanks to my children, Avery, Clara, and Adam, for reminding me daily that cribbage trumps copyediting, book reading beats blog writing, and bedtime snuggles should never be usurped by a Twitter chat.

Thank you Suzanne Digre, personal trainer, fitness writer, and editor extraordinaire, for happily reading an early draft of the first two chapters of the book and giving me fantastic and detailed feedback, not just on my writing, but on the organization of information and the details of the workout itself.

Thanks to all of my personal training clients and group fitness participants who have willingly (and sometimes unwillingly) helped me fine-tune my abilities as a trainer, instructor, and fitness writer. Having to describe and demonstrate exercises to you all on a daily basis made it much easier to write the exercise descriptions section of the book! Thanks in particular to Merrilyn Cook, Sheelagh Fitzpatrick, Jillian Freyman, Sarah Isenberg, Otilia Kozelj, Lorna Murphy, Debra Naso, Melanie Simms, Robyn Sinclair, Melody Swan, Shelley Vance, and John Harrington (my lone male client), for your ongoing interest in the book's progress and encouraging me in my debut as a fitness model.

Thanks so much to editor Lauren Harrison for doing such a fabulous job editing the original manuscript. You possess the unique combination of being able to see the big picture while still paying attention to the smallest of details. I loved that you didn't cover my writing with "red ink."

A huge thank you to my other editor Lily Chou, photographer Austin Forbord, and model Nadia Brunner-Velasquez for making the photo shoot such a fun, positive, and empowering experience. As a first time "fitness model," I had no idea what to expect from the day. Lily, your constant reminders to "suck it in" were particularly appreciated!

Thank you to my online fitness friends and colleagues Roy Cohen, Jody Goldenfield,

Deb Roby, Alexandra Williams, Kymberly Williams-Evans for filling up my Facebook feed with daily motivation, inspiration, and reminders that the health and fitness community is truly a force for positive change. Keep up the good work!

Thanks to my colleagues at the Port Moody Recreation Complex, not only for your interest in and support of my online training and writing projects, but also for willingly subbing my classes when I needed time off to write.

And finally, a heartfelt thank-you to my faithful blog readers. Without you, I would not have rediscovered my love of writing or dreamed that my words would help and motivate so many. You all inspire me daily!

About the Author

Tamara Grand lives in beautiful British Columbia, Canada, with her husband, three children, a ginger cat, and a large stash of hand-dyed yarn. She works as a BRRPA Certified Personal Trainer and Group Fitness Instructor and enjoys pushing her clients and class participants out of their comfort zones.

She is the author of the popular fitness and healthy lifestyle blog *Fitknitchick*, where she regularly shares free workouts, exercise tricks, clean eating recipes, and motivational tips. Her writing is often fueled by recent research developments in the health and fitness fields; armed with a PhD in Biology, she's uniquely capable of translating scientific jargon into language we can all understand.

Although Tamara has trained clients of all ages and fitness levels, she's particularly passionate about helping women in their 40s and 50s identify and pursue their own unique health and fitness goals. For more information about her online group training program for women over 40, please visit her website, www.fitknitchick.com.